Care to Talk

The No-Fluff OET Guide for Healthcare Professionals Who Want More Than a Pass

By Carl Halford

WARNING: PERFORMANCE AHEAD

This is not a textbook.
This is not a workbook.
This is not a friendly bundle of tips, tricks, and templates.

This is a clinical combat manual built for professionals who don't have the luxury of "just passing."
If you read this properly—and apply what it demands—
You will sound sharper.
You will write like a clinician.
You will perform like you belong in the room.

And yes—you will score higher.
Not by luck. Not by chance.
But because you trained for it like it matters.

Proceed only if:

– You're ready to leave behind "safe" English.
– You want feedback that feels like a diagnosis.
– You understand that your language is part of your clinical credibility.

If you're looking for something soft, simple, or spoon-fed—
Put this book down.

But if you're ready to speak like a leader, write like a professional, and walk into the OET like a final round interview—

Turn the page.
You're in the right place.

—The CHKZ Tactical Unit
Built for those who care to lead, not just pass.

 This badge was issued to 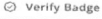 Mr Carl @ Winford International on May 11, 2023 ⊘ Verify Badge

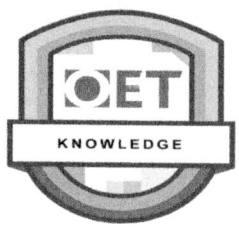

Preparation Provider: OET Knowledge

Issued by OET

The Knowledge badge covers three modules that are delivered through the Occupational English Test (OET) Preparation Provider Programme: Induction, OET Overview, and OET Knowledge. The advantage of OET (i.e. embedded in the healthcare context) and the need to improve test taking and language skills are described. The final module covers the format and skills in each sub-test and tips to help students.

Learn more

ISBN:
Published by: Self-published by Carl Halford
Cover Design by: Ms Nguyen Hanh

WHO THIS IS FOR

To my wife, Hanh (Anna), our daughter Ilithyia, and my sons, Malcolm and Alexander—
You are the reason I aim higher.
Not out of perfection, but perseverance.
I've stumbled. I've doubted. I've missed the mark.

But every lesson, every late night, and every draft of this book carried the same intent:
To build something better. For you. For us.

To the friends, colleagues, and clinicians I've had the privilege of working alongside—
From sharp nurses and radiologists to frontline doctors, vets, pathologists, forensic pathologists, pain management
specialists, radiographers, chemists, and paramedics—
You've taught me more than I've ever written down.
This book is built on your standards.
Even the ones I was closer to (in a past life, with respect)—you helped shape this too.

IF YOU'RE READY TO:

– Drop the textbook voice
– Perform under pressure
– Speak like a clinician, not a candidate

Turn the page.

The test doesn't stand a chance.
But you do.

—CHKZ
Built for those who care to lead, not just pass.

ACKNOWLEDGMENTS

No One Writes Alone.

Behind every finished book are the people who sharpened, challenged, steadied, and stood by the one writing it. This is for them.

To the clinicians who trusted me with your time, questions, frustrations, and breakthroughs—thank you for proving again and again that language is more than grammar. It's credibility. It's care. It's command. This book was sharpened by your pressure.

To the tactical minds who helped refine the structure, the tone, and the flow—thank you for calling out what didn't hit hard enough. Iron sharpens iron.

To my teaching colleagues across the years—those who've walked into staffrooms tired, underpaid, and overcommitted, yet still showed up for their learners—thank you for reminding me why precision matters.

To the students and candidates who demanded better from every lesson, task, and explanation—thank you for your high standards. This book carries your voice too.

To the mentors and medical professionals who shaped my clinical understanding, especially across emergency care, pain management, pathology radiology, and primary practice—thank you for modelling excellence under pressure.

To the healthcare professionals I've had the pleasure of knowing—some in the clinic, some in the classroom, and yes, some briefly in more personal chapters of life—thank you. You taught me where tone meets trust.

And to my inner circle—Hanh (Anna), Ilithyia, Malcolm, Alexander—you didn't just give me space to write. You gave me the reason to make it count.

Thank you for holding the line while I finished the sentence.

—Carl

EPIGRAPH

"You are never just answering a question. You are proving you belong."
– CHKZ

"Language in a clinical setting is either a scalpel or a smokescreen."
– CHKZ

"Speak as if care depends on it. Because it does."
– Adapted from frontline nursing principle

"The way you say it tells us whether to trust you."
– Paramedic Training Manual, UK NHS

"Clarity under pressure isn't a bonus. It's the job."
– CHKZ TACTICAL TRUTH

"Exams don't reward effort. They reward control."
– CHKZ

"Professionalism begins when you choose your words like tools, not feelings."
– Surgical Registrar, London Deanery

"This isn't about passing a test. It's about sounding like you already work there."
– CHKZ Candidate Briefing, Speaking Masterclass

READ THIS BEFORE YOU BLAME THE TEST

If you don't succeed with this book, it won't be because the tools weren't here.
It won't be because the language wasn't tactical, or the strategies weren't sharp.
It will be because you chose not to act.

Let's be clear.

You won't fail because:
– The material isn't ready (it is — pressure-tested and profession-proof).
– The quality isn't high enough (this is elite-level, mapped to clinical credibility, not classroom fluff).
– You don't have support (you have a vault, a system, a strategy, and the words that win under fire).
– The opportunity isn't there (every hospital, clinic, university, and visa panel demands better communicators, right now).

The only reasons you'll fail are:
– You didn't apply it.
– You didn't believe you could rise.
– You feared owning the tone of someone who belongs in the room.

That's it.

But if you do act—even modestly, even messily—this book will:

– Help you write like a clinician, not a candidate
– Help you speak like someone whose advice lands first time
– Move you from "trying to pass" to "training for leadership"
– Position you as a clinical communicator professionals want to work beside

If you fail, it's because you wanted to.
This book is the blueprint for how not to.

Choose wisely.

—CHKZ Tactical Unit
Built for professionals who treat clarity like care.

Table of Contents

FOREWORD

Dr Claire, MBBS, FRACP
Senior Consultant | Clinical Communication Lead | International Examiner

I've trained doctors who could diagnose rare syndromes in minutes—but couldn't introduce themselves without sounding unsure.
I've seen brilliant nurses write discharge letters that read like diary entries.
And I've watched good clinicians fail the OET—not because they didn't care, but because they didn't command.

This book fixes that.

Care to Talk is the resource I wish existed years ago. It doesn't explain English. It builds professionals. It rewires the way you speak, write, and show up in clinical conversations—not just to pass a test, but to lead inside it.

If you think this is just another exam prep book, think again.
This is a blueprint for sounding like someone whose words carry weight.

The first time I reviewed this material, I found myself underlining whole paragraphs—not because I'm preparing for the OET (those days are long gone)—but because even as a senior clinician and trainer, I recognised how rare it is to find a resource that blends:

– Precision and strategy
– Clinical tone and human empathy
– Psychological readiness and tactical execution

It's sharp. It's unflinching. And it holds you accountable in all the right ways.

To every healthcare professional holding this book: if your words shape decisions, guide patients, or deliver safety—this book isn't optional. It's essential.

You'll either use it—or get beaten by someone who did.

Read it. Apply it. Perform like it matters.

Because it does.

—Dr Claire
Sydney | London | Kuala Lumpur

A Note on "Originality" (Or the Clinical Truth About It)

Let's start with a clinical fact—nothing in this book is truly original.

Not the tactics.
Not the phrases.
Not even the strategies.

Language is recycled. Clinical conversations repeat. Structure follows structure.
What changes? You.

This book doesn't claim to give you some divine revelation or never-before-seen miracle method. It gives you something far more useful—a tactical system. A pressure-tested field guide. A way to sharpen how you write, speak, and show up when it counts.

Because in healthcare, there are no bonus points for originality.
There are only results. Clarity. Safety. Credibility.

Everything here is drawn from real-life clinics, real candidate struggles, real examiner feedback, and real-world performance under fire. It's the distillation of what works when the timer starts and the patient is watching—or worse, when the examiner is.

This isn't a book to passively admire.
This is a system to interact with.
Underline. Rewrite. Speak aloud. Repeat under pressure.

If you're looking for soft inspiration, this may frustrate you.
But if you're ready to dig in, challenge yourself, and train like someone who actually wants to win the job—not just scrape the score—then you're in the right hands.

Because I'm not here to inspire you. I'm here to equip you.
To provoke your thinking, structure your language, and raise your clinical performance.

So grab your pen. Flip the page. Speak like it matters.
Because it does.

—CHKZ Tactical Unit
Built for clinicians who lead through clarity.

PREFACE

Written for professionals who don't bluff. They brief.

Let me tell you why this book had to exist.

I've worked with healthcare professionals who were exceptional in the ward—but invisible on test day.
I've seen brilliant clinicians lose opportunities—not because they lacked skill, but because their communication didn't reflect it under pressure.
And I've watched too many smart, experienced candidates reduce themselves to overly polite, scripted, Band B templates—hoping to scrape through instead of commanding attention.

This book was built to stop that.

What You're Holding

Care to Talk *isn't an exam tip sheet.*
It's a tactical performance system designed for high-stakes language, delivered in high-stakes moments.

You'll learn how to:
– Speak with clinical command, not candidate hesitancy
– Write like a professional with purpose, not like a student following instructions
– Use pressure to sharpen your message, not melt your clarity
– Map every strategy to real-world care, safety, handover, and leadership

This is not for those who want a Band B and go.
This is for professionals who want their words to land—because the job, the patient, and the reputation depend on it.

Why I Wrote This

Because I've seen the difference between:
– A nurse who calms a patient with 8 words instead of 80
– A doctor who delivers instructions the first time—clearly, precisely
– A radiologist who writes a letter that sounds like authority, not ambiguity

And I've watched them all struggle with OET prep materials that water down what makes them brilliant.

I wanted to give them something sharper.
Something worthy of their profession.
Something that doesn't train you to sound like a textbook—but like someone already in the job.

If You're Still Reading

Good.

Because this book will demand effort.
It will challenge how you speak. How you write. How you frame your thoughts.
But it will also raise your standard—and give you the tools to reach it.

This book won't just get you the score.
It'll get you heard. Respected. Remembered.

Now let's begin.

—Carl
Clinical trainer, language strategist, and the guy who refuses to let good clinicians fail on paper.

What Is an OET Trainer, Really?

And Who Are All These Brilliant (and Occasionally Bizarre) Humans Who Call Themselves One?

Let's cut the clinical fluff.

An OET trainer isn't just someone with a headset mic and a copy of the sample test.
They're a translator of tone. A strategist of speech. A sculptor of clarity.
They live at the crossroads of medicine and language—and they know a single preposition can be the difference between safe care and catastrophic confusion.

But let's be honest: not all OET trainers are the same.
Some arrived here through medicine. Some through English. Some through a chaotic fusion of both.
They're spread across clinics, classrooms, backroom Zoom calls, IELTS centres, hospital basements, and side gigs that somehow became full-time empires.

Here are just a few you might recognise:

1. The Clinical Insider

Former nurse. Current communication weapon.
Knows how to hold a stethoscope, fill in a discharge letter, and spot tone errors faster than a spellcheck.
Fluent in both SOAP notes and patient-centred empathy.
They don't teach OET—they live it.

2. The Grammar Jedi

Can break down relative clauses like surgical anatomy.
Carries a mini whiteboard to coffee shops just in case.
Has a love–hate relationship with passive voice.
Says things like, "Let's restructure for conciseness," in casual conversation.

3. The IELTS Veteran Turned Convert

They've marked enough Task 2 essays to fill a warehouse.
Now they're here, breathing a sigh of relief every time a candidate actually has a purpose for writing.
They still twitch when someone says "coherence and cohesion," but they've found new life in role-play drills.

4. The Medical Spouse

Didn't study medicine—just married it.
Knows more about discharge planning and wound care than most first year residents.
Teaches OET by osmosis and lived experience.
Their superpower? Translating doctor-speak into Band A performance.

5. The Night-Shift Language Warrior

Teaches OET after dark, between two hospital shifts or one too many admin emails.
They run crash courses, survival drills, and pep talks at 10 p.m.

Armed with caffeine, PowerPoint, and pure belief.

6. The Clinical Drama Coach

Has a background in acting, coaching, or trauma-informed education.
Teaches tone like it's theatre, and role-plays like it's Broadway.
Fierce on vocal delivery. Ruthless on pauses.
Believes speaking tests are performances—and trains you to own the stage.

7. The Expat Educator

From Bangkok to Bucharest, they've taught OET in basements, clinics, cafés, and broom cupboards.
They've hauled grammar books across continents, run crash courses in hotel lobbies, and know which embassies give the fastest certification letters.
They're not training for a job. They're training for a calling.

8. The Plug-and-Play Trainer-Turned-Entrepreneur

Used this book as a base, built a programme, and now runs a micro-empire.
They offer mock tests, feedback clinics, group intensives, and private Band A coaching—with clinical partners on speed dial.
They sell clarity. And their students pass.

So… What Is an OET Trainer?

An OET trainer is part coach, part clinician, part linguist, part therapist.
They're a walking, talking filter for what lands with patients, what scores with examiners, and what keeps healthcare professionals from playing small.

If you're reading this book, chances are you're one of them.

So let's say this clearly:

Whether you came through nursing, TESOL, coaching, linguistics, or pure survival…
Whether you wear scrubs or a hoodie…
Whether you're Band A certified or still finding your feet…

You belong here.

Because if you're helping professionals care better through communication,
you're not just teaching English.
You're training clarity.
You're protecting patients.
You're changing careers—and sometimes lives.

Welcome to Care to Talk.
Let's train like it matters.
Because it does.

Training Outstanding OET Speaking Lessons

From "Good Enough" to "Clinically Commanding" in the High-Stakes English Arena

So - You've got a role-play card, a clinical scenario, a group of nurses, doctors, or healthcare workers in front of you—and one unspoken hope in their eyes:

"Please don't make me feel small today."

Outstanding OET speaking lessons aren't about charisma, colourful whiteboards, or clever grammar explanations. They're about preparing clinicians to speak under pressure with clarity, control, and clinical credibility—even when their brain is tired, their accent is strong, and the timer is ticking.

This section is your complete tactical kitbag for doing exactly that.

What Makes an OET Speaking Lesson Outstanding?
Let's strip it back. A top-tier lesson trains your candidates to:
Say what they mean
Mean what they say
Say it clearly, confidently, and clinically—especially in real-world, high-stakes moments

We do this by building:
Language Input: function-rich, context-tied phrases
Controlled Practice: safe space, clear tasks, scaffolding
Communicative Output: messy, realistic, and self-aware performance

All layered with:
Repetition
Role variation
Clinical simulation
Meta-cognitive reflection
Tactical feedback

Golden Rule:
"If they're talking more than you—good.
If they're talking with purpose, structure, and real-world relevance—excellent."

Core Strategies for Outstanding OET Speaking Training

1. Start with a Situation, Not a Sub-Skill
Don't say:
"Today we'll practise empathy."

Say:
"You're the night nurse. The Patient's angry. The meds are delayed. What do you say?"

Why it works:
Situation triggers urgency. Urgency builds strategy. Strategy under pressure = performance.

2. Teach Phrases That Survive Under Pressure

Don't teach "apologise" in isolation.

Teach:
"I do apologise for the delay."
"Thank you for your patience—I know it's frustrating."
"Let me check that for you right now."

Phrase = control.
Chunk = fluency.
Real-life = retention.

3. Model Before They Perform

Use demos:
Video clips
Audio strips
Annotated transcripts
Trainer live role-play

EXAMINER TRIGGER POINT: If they've never heard what a Band A tone sounds like, they can't replicate it. Model everything—pacing, empathy, transitions, and close.

4. Repetition Without Redundancy

Change the emotion. Shift the setting. Rotate the role.

Try this sequence:
Scenario: confused Patient
Repetition: now the Patient is angry
New speaker: switch to Admin role
New task: now it's explaining vs. apologising
Repetition = familiarity
Variation = resilience

5. Visual Prompts > Verbal Panic

Use:
Scenario cards
Picture cues (medications, masks, signage)
Setting maps (ward, desk, triage room)
Task flashcards
Emotion tags
Visuals reduce mental load. They keep focus on function, not vocabulary panic.

6. Sentence Starters = Confidence Triggers

Give them the launch pad:
"Let me reassure you that…"
"It's completely normal to feel…"
"Can I confirm a few details before we proceed?"
"Please let me know if anything feels unclear."

Pair with:
Roles: Nurse, Doctor, Radiologist, Admin
Emotions: Nervous, Frustrated, Grateful, Scared
This turns "just speaking" into clinical communication.

7. Build Real Pressure in a Safe Space
Balance urgency + safety:
2-minute countdown challenges
Peer feedback scorecards (1 win + 1 upgrade)
Voice/video recordings for playback
Tactical Debrief: "What worked? What failed under stress?"
Create a culture where mistakes are drills, not defeats.

CHKZ TRAINER TOOLS FOR SURVIVAL & SUCCESS

Tactic	Why It Works
Write great student phrases on the board as they say them	Reinforces their own success live
Shadow native audio strips	Boosts pacing, rhythm, and stress pattern confidence
Freeze & Fix	**Mid-role-play pause:** "Could we improve that line?"
"Walk & Talk" rounds	Builds fluency while reducing performance anxiety
Let them choose feedback focus	**Empowers ownership:** Pronunciation / Tone / Transitions

Real-World Simulation Example
Task: "Explain a Delay and Reassure the Patient"
Input:
Vocabulary: delay, appointment, apologise, reassure, unexpected
Phrases: "I appreciate your patience." / "There's been a delay with the lab."
Tone: Calm, empathetic, authoritative
Practice:
Fill-in-the-gap dialogue (controlled)
Role-play (Patient emotion: angry → anxious)
Timed explanations with scorecard feedback
Output:
Final simulation with rotation roles
Reflection: "Did I explain clearly? Did I own the tone?"

Final Words to OET Speaking Trainers
Fluency isn't perfection.
Fluency is professional clarity spoken under pressure—with calm, care, and confidence.
Your job isn't just to get them speaking.
It's to help them believe they belong in the conversation.

Even when their grammar isn't flawless. Even when the timer starts.
Even when they feel like an outsider in the system.

Because when they walk into that exam—and into their next ward, interview, or OSCE—
They won't just be "candidates."
They'll sound like clinicians.

Because you trained them to.

—CHKZ
Where speaking isn't small talk. It's clinical command.

Understanding Your OET Candidates

They're Not Just Candidates. They're Clinicians With Careers, Chaos, and Courage.

Let's get one thing clear:

OET candidates are not test-takers with empty notebooks and spare weekends.

They are working professionals. Real humans. Often exhausted, overcommitted, and quietly carrying the weight of career migration, family pressure, and clinical responsibility.

They are not here for a grammar class.
They are here because their future depends on their ability to speak and write under pressure—with clarity, control, and care.

Your job?

Not to "teach a lesson."
But to build belief and tactical confidence in the limited time you've got.

Who's Actually in Your OET Room?
A nurse straight off a 12-hour shift who barely had time to eat
A lab technician whose visa depends on this next exam
A radiologist with perfect passive voice… and paralysing speaking anxiety
A mother juggling night shifts, teething toddlers, and Band B stress
A healthcare admin who knows the vocabulary—but not how to use it under fire
A senior doctor trying to relocate their family across continents and systems

These are not lazy learners.
They are living on the edge of everything. And they've chosen to show up.

Sometimes that means:
– They're late (because the bus didn't come or the ward handover overran)
– They forget homework (because they slept three hours)
– They freeze mid-sentence (because their brain is in Tagalog, Arabic, or French mode)
– They cry after class (because they haven't seen their family in six months)
This isn't a language class. This is a life upgrade under pressure.

Golden Ratio: Candidate Talk Time > Trainer Talk Time
If you're speaking more than them, they're not improving.
You're not the star. They are.

Outstanding trainers engineer lessons where:
– You ask more than you explain
– You set up tasks, not lectures
– You elicit phrases, not silence
– You listen for tone, not just tenses

Because this isn't about grammar perfection.
It's about survival-grade fluency, structure, and control in real-world scenarios.

"But What If They Struggle?"

They will.
That's not failure. That's training.
Your job isn't to protect them from mistakes.

It's to create an environment where making one doesn't shatter their credibility.
Instead of finishing their sentence—scaffold it.
Instead of correcting everything—focus on clarity and tone.
Instead of jumping in—pause, wait, hold the space.

Give them the tools to survive a sentence breakdown:

"Let me rephrase that."
"What I mean is…"
"Can I explain that a different way?"
You're not teaching English.
You're teaching linguistic resilience.

Pronunciation: The Silent Shame They Carry
They know the word "anaphylaxis."
But they fear saying it will cost them their score—or worse, their dignity.

Drill the words that cause self-doubt:

Stress patterns: "IN-jection," not "in-JEC-tion"
Rhythm chunks: "Let-me-check-for-you" not "Let. Me. Check."
Critical terms: "hypertension," "prescription," "emergency," "allergic reaction"

Reminder: Clarity breeds confidence.
And confidence changes tone.
And tone changes perception.
And perception changes whether they pass—or get passed over.

Not Every Learner Enters at the Same Gate

In every session, you'll find:

Learner Type	Strategy
Slow Processors	Visual prompts. Repeat drills. Give wait time.
High-Flyers	Leadership roles. Peer modelling. Add time pressure.
Grammar Analysts	Set a "grammar parking lot." Return later. Keep pace.
Quiet but Capable	One-to-one warm-ups. Partner tasks before group drills.
Fast Talkers with Chaos	Give frameworks. Score structure. Don't reward speed alone.

Your job isn't to treat everyone equally.
It's to treat everyone fairly.
And that means giving each candidate what they need to perform under fire.

Trainer's Toolkit: Meeting Learners Where They Are

Challenge	Tactical Response
Nervous Speakers	Pair work. Starter scripts. Safe warm-ups.
Confident But Messy	Task-based peer feedback. Tone-target drills.
Silent Thinkers	Prep time. Personal notes. Think–Pair–Share.
Emotionally Overwhelmed	Breathing breaks. Recap cycles. Reset opportunities.
Natural Leaders	Let them mentor. Showcase them as models.

Final Words for OET Trainers
Your candidates won't remember:
– Your slides
– Your board layout
– The perfect CEFR term for "discourse markers"

But they will remember:
– That you didn't make them feel stupid
– That you believed they could sound like a professional
– That they finally said something right—and didn't feel ashamed

You can't fix their visa stress.
You can't give them more time or energy.
You can't speed up learning like a Netflix binge.

But you can build a space where adults under pressure find a voice worth listening to.

Where they become clinicians who sound like they belong.

And that's what makes you a trainer worth trusting.

—CHKZ
Where communication is clinical. And clarity is care.

The OET Trainer in the Room

Your Presence. Their Performance. The Standard You Set.

Let's strip it down.

You can walk in with perfect handouts, well-aligned slides, and a laminated scheme of work —
but if you show up unfocused, unconvincing, or unprepared to lead, it all falls apart before the second role-play begins.

OET candidates don't just learn from your worksheets.
They learn from your tone. Your posture. Your control. Your clarity under pressure.

You're not just delivering content.
You're modelling clinical communication under fire.

This section is your trainer reset.
Not to be perfect — but to be present, professional, and performance-focused in every room you enter.

1. Be Early. Because Late Is a Leadership Leak.
Arriving late tells the room:
– You're not ready.
– This doesn't matter.
– Neither do they.

Arriving early tells the room:
– I'm calm.
– You're worth preparing for.
– Let's work at Band A level from the first second.
Set up the room. Test the AV. Mentally rehearse.
Your calm is built. Not borrowed.

2. Know the Plan. Lead With Precision.
OET training is clinical. Timed. Tactical.

Before you say a word, know:
– What sub-skills you're targeting
– How today's drills map to criteria
– What every activity earns them under pressure
You're not "just doing Speaking Part B."
You're engineering performance improvements with professional consequences.
Plan the next 10 minutes like it's an OSCE station. Because for them — it might as well be.

3. Your Tone Sets the Temperature.
You want them to be focused, respectful, responsive?
Start with you.
– Speak with control.
– Move with purpose.
– Greet them like professionals, not students.
– Hold space like someone who runs a clinic, not a club.

Your voice becomes their standard. Your posture becomes their template.

4. Feedback Isn't Flattery. It's Fuel.
Effective OET feedback is:
– **Timely**: Today's errors addressed today
– **Tactical**: Mapped to criteria, not feelings
– **Specific**: "Your reassurance line hit perfectly — calm tone, clear phrase"
– **Balanced**: Reinforce what worked, reframe what didn't

Bonus: Use peer feedback and self-assessment tools. Build professional self-awareness. Train clinicians to listen like examiners.

5. Be There. Fully. No Drift.
Scrolling mid-task? Daydreaming during a role-play?
You just downgraded the room to Band C.

Instead:
– Listen with intent
– Watch tone, word choice, body language
– Ask real follow-ups
– Give eye contact that says, You're being assessed, but not judged
Presence is what separates a trainer from a talker.

6. Speak Like a Clinician. Train Like It Matters.
You're not a game show host.
You're not a grammar guru.

You are:
– A performance coach
– A tone strategist
– A leadership model
Use real-life examples.
Share clinical analogies.
Show what it sounds like when someone walks into the OET already sounding like they belong there.
If you're boring, they switch off.
If you're compelling, they step up.

7. Link Motivation to Mission.
Skip the fluff.
Don't just say, "You've got this!"

Say:
"Every sentence you improve sharpens your professional identity."
"This phrase gives you power in your next ward shift."
"When you say it like that, they'll believe you."
Motivation doesn't come from cheerleading.
It comes from connection to consequences.

8. Politeness Is Not Optional. It's Professional Modelling.

You want Band A tone? Model it.

– Say thank you.

– Ask, not demand.

– Correct with clinical calm, not classroom sarcasm.

– Never mock. Never shame.

This isn't about being "nice."

It's about teaching them how to speak to patients, colleagues, examiners, and employers — with empathy, structure, and respect.

9. **Read the Room. Adapt Like a Leader.**

Who's withdrawing?

Who's dominating?

Who's misunderstanding the task criteria?

Who's ready to upgrade?

Now pivot.

– Change the pairings

– Reassign roles

– Adjust the timing

– Clarify the task

Great trainers don't run lessons.

They run diagnostics mid-flight and adjust in real time.

10. **Reflect Like a Clinician.**

After every session, ask:

– What improved?

– Who still needs a breakthrough?

– Did I hold the room?

– Did I model Band A?

Keep a short, sharp trainer log.

Note names. Highlight patterns. Track tone progression.

Teaching is performance coaching.

Not delivery. Not discussion.

It's clinical calibration—one learner at a time.

Final Note: You Are the Exam Room Before the Exam Room

You are:

– The first examiner they face

– The voice in their head under pressure

– The model they mirror when they panic

So be the professional you'd want next to you when it counts.

Be early.

Be precise.

Be composed.

Be respectful.

Be unshakeable.

You don't need to be perfect.

But if you're consistent, clear, and commanding—

They'll walk into that test room already transformed.

—CHKZ
Built for trainers who create clinicians, not just candidates.

OET Lesson Preparation & Management

This Isn't a Class. It's a Simulation. Own the Room Like a Clinical Lead.

Let's be blunt:
You could have flawless slides.
You could have a role-play that's examiner-approved, rubric-aligned, and beautifully scaffolded.

But if your room is distracted, disjointed, or running on fumes — it won't land.
Not the task. Not the tone. Not the transformation.

OET lesson management isn't about being liked.
It's about being clear, calm, and clinically commanding.

This isn't a high school English room.
This is a high-stakes language pressure lab—where confidence, credibility, and clarity are built under pressure.

1. Authority Is a Clinical Vibe, Not a Volume Level
You don't walk in as "just a teacher."
You walk in as the language leader of the shift.

Respect is earned by:
– Being early
– Being calm
– Speaking with structured clarity
– Holding boundaries without apology
Don't beg for attention.
Don't repeat instructions like it's karaoke.
Speak once. Speak well. Let the silence do the rest.

Trainer Command Code:
"Be precise. Be calm. Be the adult in the room when the pressure hits."

2. Routines Reduce Stress. Build Them Relentlessly.
The best OET trainers don't improvise their entry. They ritualise it.

Set routines that train professionalism:
– Clinical-style greeting: direct, calm, "Good to see you. Let's begin."
– Warm-up task visible and running the moment they arrive
– Time-boxed objectives written, stated, and repeated
– Lesson ends with recap, reflection, and next-step activation
Predictability = safety.
Safety = confidence.
Confidence = better performance under exam pressure.

3. Talk Less. Deliver More.
Dump the TED Talk. They didn't pay for a monologue.

Instead:
– Chunk instructions
– Use gesture and clinical examples
– Confirm with "What will you do first?" instead of "Any questions?"
– Pause long enough for thinking
– Give sentence stems like "Let me clarify that…" / "Can I confirm…"
The trainer isn't the centre. The speaking candidate is.

4. Use Your Presence Like a Senior Clinician

Don't manage with volume. Manage with gravity.
– Stand still when giving instructions
– Walk the room like you own it
– Pause deliberately
– Use direct eye contact to anchor attention
– Park yourself silently near off-task groups—no words needed
You're not a disciplinarian. You're a presence.
And presence under pressure is what they're being trained to copy.

5. Build Systems That Lead, Not Noise That Chases

Raise your hand? They stop.
Silent countdown? They reset.
Off-task? They know the routine response.
Need help? They signal without breaking the task.
System > shouting.
Routine > reminders.
Structure > stress.
If you're managing chaos with noise, you're late to your own intervention.

6. Anticipate Friction. Don't Chase It.

Great trainers don't put out fires. They remove the matches.

Watch for:
– Group confusion = clarify task BEFORE they dive in
– Volume creeping = insert a timed mini-drill to refocus
– Someone faking fluency = throw in cold prompts, not corrections
Stay one beat ahead. That's how surgeons work. That's how trainers win.

7. Define Roles to Eliminate Drift

Group role-play? Role it properly.

Assign:
– The Speaker
– The Accuracy Checker
– The Timekeeper
– The Observer
Clarity kills confusion.
Defined roles kill dominance.
No one floats. Everyone performs.
This mirrors the team-based structure of healthcare—and reinforces responsibility under structure.

8. Correct the Behaviour, Not the Person

When someone's off-task, don't lecture. Don't belittle.

"You always ignore instructions."

"Let's pause — phones down, focus back here. We're running this drill together."

Correct the action, not the identity.

You're modelling professional interaction—whether they know it or not.

9. Remember: They're Not Students. They're Clinicians Under Pressure.

Yes, some are late.

Yes, some forget their phrases.

Yes, some speak too little or too much or not at all.

But they are:
– Parents
– Migrants
– Professionals
– Survivors of burnout
– Humans betting their next chapter on this test

So:
– Be kind, but firm.
– Be professional, not performative.
– Be the one person in their week who holds the line without shaming them for struggling to walk it.

Final Word: You Are the First Simulation

The way you manage the lesson is the way they learn to manage their clinical voice.

You're not just setting up activities.

You're setting up a standard of performance.

Be structured.
Be strategic.
Be steady.
Be sharp.

The lesson isn't the experience.
You are.

—CHKZ
This isn't classroom management. This is clinical leadership rehearsal.

The Power of an OET Lesson Plan

Real Performance Doesn't Happen by Accident. It's Engineered. Strategically. Clinically. Relentlessly.

Behind every confident Band A speaker...
Behind every upgraded writing sample...
Behind every clinician who finally says,

"I know how to say this — and say it well,"
there's a lesson plan.

Not a scribbled note on a napkin.
Not a recycled worksheet with new headings.
But a real plan. A performance blueprint.
Clear. Tactical. Built to hold under pressure.

What Is an OET Lesson Plan?

It's not admin. It's not paperwork.
It's not a tick-box to show your boss you did "something."
A lesson plan is a mission brief —
Your strategy for turning stress-prone candidates into structured communicators.

A great OET lesson plan answers:

– What sub-skills are we building today?
– What professional behaviours are we rehearsing?
– How will I support the hesitant... and challenge the high-flyers?
– Where does this connect to clinical safety, tone, or trust?
This book doesn't give you theory.
It gives you working tools.
Plans built by trainers, refined with candidates, and sharpened under real test pressure.

What's Inside Each Tactical Plan?
Every CHKZ lesson plan is:

– OET Criteria-Aligned (so you're always building towards scoring reality)
– CEFR-Mapped (so progression has a spine)
– Function-Based (because "accuracy" without clinical purpose is just noise)
– Tone-Aware (because how you say it earns just as many points as what you say)
– Flexible (adaptable for role-play, workshops, clinics, or 1:1 performance sessions)

Expect:

Language input that matters under fire
Output tasks that simulate real scenarios
Built-in differentiation (because not all candidates need the same drill)
Reflection prompts (because growth starts with self-awareness)

Why Even Experienced Trainers Still Plan
If you've been teaching OET for years, this might be your inner voice:

"I don't need a lesson plan. I've got experience."
But let's reframe that.

Surgeons still follow protocols.
Pilots still run pre-flight checks.
Clinicians still prepare before a ward round.
Why?
BECAUSE WHEN THE STAKES ARE HIGH — STRUCTURE PROTECTS PERFORMANCE.

A real plan ensures:
– Focus under pressure
– Clear transitions between input and output
– No drift, no dead-time, no wasted effort
– You're building skills that actually land in the test room
No more recycled filler.
No more "see how it goes."
You're not filling time. You're forging control.

Plans That Perform — Even When You Step Out
A well-designed OET lesson plan doesn't just help you teach.
It allows another trainer to walk in, pick it up, and deliver with consistency and care.

Why that matters:
– In clinics, language precision = patient safety
– In teams, trainer alignment = candidate trust
– In preparation centres, clarity = long-term credibility

This book's plans are designed for:
– Rapid deployment
– Mixed-level groups
– Simulation-heavy sessions
– Trainer rotation and handover

Final Word: A Plan Is Not Paperwork. It's Precision.
When you plan well, you don't just run a 90-minute session.
You build confidence. You train tone. You rehearse authority.

Each plan in this book is:
– Clinically relevant
– Culturally attuned
– Professionally ambitious
– Built to win under pressure

Whether you're teaching a newcomer, running an intensive, or delivering CPD for clinical staff—
Let the plan lead. Then adapt it with purpose.

Because lesson planning is not bureaucracy.

It's clinical leadership in linguistic form.

—CHKZ
Built for trainers who turn plans into performance.

DURING THE LESSON

Where Pressure Meets Performance — And You Guide the Shift

There's what's on paper…
And then there's what happens when real humans walk in — tired, nervous, overqualified, and underconfident.

One is a plan.
The other is a live simulation of future clinical conversations — compressed into 90 minutes of high-stakes language training.

You've prepped. You've printed. You've planned the drill.

Now it's game time.
This isn't just a lesson.
This is performance rehearsal under pressure — and you're the one running the room.

1. **Move With Intention. Not Distraction**.
Don't pace like a monitor.
Move like a mentor.
– Walk the room with quiet purpose
– Join a pair momentarily, then drift
– Sit next to someone struggling
– Observe tone shifts, not just grammar slips

Your movement communicates:
– "You're being seen"
– "I care how you're performing"
– "This is a professional environment"
Close enough to support.
Far enough to respect space.
Present enough to read the unsaid.

2. **Ditch "Do You Understand?" Forever**
"Do you understand?" guarantees a polite nod — and silent confusion.

Use ICQs to confirm instructions:
"Are we writing full sentences or bullet points?"
"How long do you have?"
"Alone or in pairs?"

Use CCQs to confirm comprehension:
"If something's urgent, should you wait?" → No
"If you say, 'Let me reassure you,' are you warning or calming?" → Calming
"Is 'I'll get back to you' a promise or a delay?" → Context matters
This isn't ESL. It's language for liability, clarity, and care. Ask better.

3. **Feedback Must Be Live, Light, and Laser-Focused**
Feedback shouldn't wait until "after class."

– Correct in motion
– Highlight strong phrases in real-time

– Use the 3-Error Rule: Don't flood. Fix what matters
Focus on:
– Message clarity
– Clinical tone
– Phrase-level structure

Say:
"Excellent use of reassurance — calm tone and functional phrasing."

Not:
"Good job." (What job?)
Feedback is a diagnostic, not a compliment.

4. Praise With Precision
Praise isn't motivation. It's modelling.

Don't say:
"Nice work!"

Say:
"That line — 'Let me double-check that for you' — hit the exact tone we want under pressure."
Your praise should build repeatable behaviours.
Don't reward correctness.
Reward clinical control.

5. Turn Learners Into Evaluators
You're not their only feedback source.

Train them to:
– Review each other's role-plays
– Spot clarity gaps
– Score tone, empathy, and control

Ask:
– "What phrase really worked?"
– "What would make that message stronger?"
– "Would you feel reassured as the patient?"

This builds:
– Self-regulation
– Peer respect
– Real-world reflection
And it removes the myth that only "the trainer" knows what's right.

6. Pause the Clock. Process the Performance.

After every output task:
– Debrief
– Reflect
– Anchor the win

Ask:
"What helped you sound more confident?"
"Where did it start to fall apart — and why?"
"What will you try differently next time?"
This isn't a classroom. It's a clinic of communication.
Let them operate — then reflect on what worked, what didn't, and what evolves next.

7. Inject Energy With Tactical Micro-Drills
Keep attention sharp with fast bursts of intensity:
– "Repeat after me" – for rhythm and tone
– "Describe this without using the word" – for fluency stretch
– "Quickfire reassurances – 4 in 30 seconds"
– "Stand up if you can spot the tone error"
These are small drills with big return.
No slides. No prep.
Just linguistic combat training in motion.

8. Use Tech to Simulate Real-World Tools
Don't just "teach OET." Teach survival.
– Use Google to find real signage
– Watch clinical dialogues with subtitles
– Use voice-to-text tools to review pacing and pronunciation
– Record role-plays and self-score using criteria
– Search terms live to build self-correction reflexes
Tech in the OET room isn't distraction.
It's preparation for a digitally literate medical world.

9. Know When to Get Out of the Way
You've prepped the simulation. Now let it run.
– Set up the task
– Clarify the roles
– Step back and watch the test rehearsal begin

Don't fill every silence.
Don't over-model.
Don't hover like a lifeguard.

Let them speak.
Let them struggle.
Let them discover how they perform under pressure.

You're not the hero.
You're the guide who disappears at the right moment.

Final Word: The Lesson Isn't the Magic — You Are
In those 90 minutes, you're not just teaching.

You're:
– A mirror (reflecting back potential)
– A coach (shaping performance)
– A clinician of communication (modelling what good sounds like)
– A leader under fire

OET success is earned during these moments — not from tips, not from textbooks, not from luck.

Show up sharp.

Train like it matters.

Let them walk out sounding like professionals.

Because they will only believe they can — if you model what belief sounds like.

—CHKZ
This isn't classroom time. This is clinical command in training.

HOW TO USE THIS BOOK

This Isn't a Textbook. It's a Tactical Upgrade System.

Let's be clinically clear.
This book was not designed to be read passively.
It was engineered to be applied, rehearsed, and performed under pressure.
Think of it as a training manual, not a reading task.

You don't browse this book.
You deploy it.

Whether you're preparing as a candidate, delivering as a trainer, or rebuilding your Band B learners from the ground up—this book gives you:

System-level clarity on every OET component
Profession-specific drills for performance
Phrase-level upgrades to sound more credible
Psychological tools to handle the pressure
And a trainer-mode track for teaching it all with authority

Structure Breakdown
This book is built in 8 Parts and supported by Toolkits, Tracks, and Vault Access.

Each chapter is:
– Aligned to OET sub-tests and official criteria
– Layered with CHKZ tactical framing
– Embedded with Band A strategies under time pressure
– Designed to apply across all 12 OET professions

You'll also find:
Mindset reframes to shift you from "test taker" to clinical communicator
Live trainer notes to coach others using the book
QR Vault links to unlock drills, walkthroughs, and audio examples
By-band pathways to help you know exactly where to enter and how to grow

Choose Your Track. Start Where You Need.

This is not a cover-to-cover journey unless you want it to be. Use the entry pathways mapped out inside.

Goal	Start Here
Speaking only	Chapters 5–8 → Role-Play Set → Appendix A1 / A2
Writing focus	Chapters 9–12 → Task Set → Appendix A3 / A7
Listening sharpener	Chapter 20 → Drill Zone → Appendix A6
Full Band A system	Begin at Chapter 1. Follow it through. Apply as you go.
Trainer mode	Watch for margin icons + see Trainer Rubric in Appendix A2

Goal	Start Here
Survival kit	Flip to Part 7: Practice & Pressure Tasks

Every chapter includes:
– Component breakdown
– Band A targets
– Strategy scripts and examples
– real-world transfer prompts
– Tactical drills to apply immediately

Key Symbols & Tools Inside
Look out for:
• **CLINICIAN'S CHOICE** – Optional phrase or strategy for extra clinical precision
• **PHRASES THAT WIN POINTS** – Drop-in chunks designed to boost score and tone
• **EXAMINER TRIGGER POINTS** – Where candidates typically lose marks under pressure
• **TACTICAL TRUTHs** – CHKZ reframes that shift thinking fast
• **STRATEGIC ERROR Alerts** – Band B traps you must avoid

You'll also find:
– By-Profession Tags: so every nurse, doctor, pharmacist, or physio sees themselves in the content
– CEFR–OET Mapping: see how your growth aligns with both scales
– Trainer Differentiation Notes: instant up/down-scaling strategies built in

For Trainers: How to Use This Book in the Field
This is your ready-to-run system:
Use chapters as standalone CPD or course units

Print selected drills for 1:1 or group intensives
Use Trainer Strip notes for on-the-fly feedback
Set reading targets for independent learner follow-up
Build internal mock tests using the tasks and rubrics provided
Plug in Vault audio links during class for simulations
This book was designed to make OET teaching trainer-proof — not because trainers can't teach, but because structure builds scale and impact.

For Candidates: How to Make It Count
Read one chapter.
Apply the drills.
Speak the phrases out loud.
Write the structures by hand.
Use a mirror. Use a voice recorder. Use a friend. Just don't read and walk away.

The fastest growth happens when you:
– Say what you've learned
– Use it in role-play
– Record, reflect, and retry
– Drill under pressure, not in comfort
– Think like a clinician. Speak like one too.

Final Note: This Book Has a Vault.
Literally.

Throughout the book, you'll find QR codes and Vault entry points. These unlock:
– Audio simulations
– Drill packs
– Printable phrase banks
– Speaking models
– Reflection sheets
– Trainer assets and briefings

Use the book. Then unlock the vault. Because what you apply is what changes your performance — not what you highlight.

CHKZ FINAL BRIEFING

This isn't a book. It's a performance upgrade system.
You're not just a reader. You're the clinician in training.
Read. Drill. Reflect. Upgrade. Lead.

Let's begin.

—CHKZ
Where English meets leadership. And clarity becomes care.

INTRODUCTION

This Isn't Just About a Test. It's About How You're Heard — When It Counts.

Let's get something straight.
The OET isn't just a language test.
It's a credibility test.
It measures how well you speak, write, listen, and read under pressure—but more than that, it reveals how ready you are to sound like someone who belongs in the job.

If that sounds harsh, good. This book was not built to make you feel safe. It was built to make you ready. Because in healthcare, language isn't decoration.

It's delivery.
It's trust.
It's safety.

And in an exam where a single phrase can shift the tone from "student" to "clinician," you need more than test tips. You need performance strategy.

Why This Book Matters
You don't rise to the level of your hopes.
You rise to the level of your preparation.

Care to Talk exists for one reason:
To help healthcare professionals—from nurses and doctors to dentists, physios, pharmacists, vets, and more—train for high-impact communication in both the test room and the real world.

This book is:
– Clinically aligned
– Psychologically framed
– Strategically built
– Professionally respected
And above all — honest.
No padding. No soft encouragement.
Just the tools, scripts, drills, mindsets, and models that get you results.

Who This Book Is For
– Healthcare professionals chasing Band A
– Band B survivors ready to go higher
– OET trainers who want to coach with structure, not stress
– Medical educators tired of generic ESL methods
– Candidates who don't want to just pass — they want to own the room

Whether you're a junior doctor navigating visa deadlines, a nurse preparing for a registration panel, or a speech pathologist switching systems, this book was built with you in mind.

What You'll Get Inside

– Tactical breakdowns of each OET component
– Profession-by-profession models and tasks
– Phrase banks and strategy scripts
– CEFR–OET crosswalks
– Trainer tools and pressure-proof drills
– Digital Vault access for simulations and feedback kits
– Psychological tools for clarity, confidence, and control
This isn't about sounding perfect.
It's about sounding professional—with tone, purpose, and leadership.

Why Now?
Because OET isn't getting easier.
Because your competitors aren't waiting.
Because hospitals, clinics, and universities are choosing based on how you communicate—not just your qualifications.
And because you deserve to be in the room, not just hoping to get through the door.

So welcome to the system.

The no-fluff, no-shortcut, high-standard way to speak like it matters, and lead like you belong.

Let's get to work.

—CHKZ
Built for those who care to talk. And talk to care.

Care to Talk

PART 1 – THE ARENA

Know the Game. Play to Win.

Before you step into the test room, you need to understand something most candidates never do:

This isn't an exam. It's an audition.
You're not here to "use English."
You're here to prove clinical command through the way you speak, write, respond, and lead under pressure.

The OET is not a vocabulary quiz.
It's a credibility filter.

Every phrase you say, every line you write, every pause you hold — tells the examiner whether they'd trust you with a real patient, in a real clinic, under real fire.

Welcome to the Arena.

This part of the book will reshape how you see the OET — not as a paper-based performance, but as a tactical landscape that requires strategy, structure, and psychological edge. No fluff. No guesswork. Just clarity, control, and career-grade communication.

Here's What You're About to Walk Into:
Chapter 1 – The Stakes Are Higher Than Just a Pass
This chapter hits hard, fast, and honest. It's not about scaring you.
It's about waking you up.
What happens if you settle for Band B?
What's the real cost — in time, visas, contracts, career progression, or personal belief?
We expose the Band B trap, reframe the mission, and show you why your language isn't "just English" — it's your professional signature.
Trainer Trigger: "What's the cost of staying average?"

Chapter 2 – Decoding the OET Battlefield
The map. The mechanics. The mission.
This chapter breaks the test into what it really is — a timed pressure system across four performance zones.

We'll walk you through:
– How the scoring really works
– What the examiners are trained to listen for
– Where most candidates burn time and points
– And how to flip test-day nerves into trained execution
Includes: "Visual OET Command Map" + time-pressure matrix

Chapter 3 – The 12 Professions, One Standard
Whether you're a nurse or a dentist, a vet or a physio — the bar is the same: communicate like a clinician.
This chapter shows you:
– What's universal across all 12 professions

– What's unique in tone, function, or format
– How to filter your prep for your field
– How to spot and adopt the shared language of clinical credibility
Profession icons + QR-linked Vault bonuses by job role

Chapter 4 – Textbook English vs Tactical English
Here's the cold truth:
You can speak perfect English… and still sound like a Band B candidate.
This chapter exposes the gap between safe language and scoring language.
We dissect weak phrasing, over-politeness, robotic transitions, and misused tone.
You'll learn what Band A actually sounds like when the pressure is real.
Includes: Examiner Red Flag Callouts — phrases that cost points fast

What Part I Will Give You
Total clarity on what OET really measures
Tactical awareness of what can win or lose marks
A mindset shift — from passive prep to pressure performance
Strategic prep entry points no one else teaches
Profession-specific awareness to avoid generic coaching traps

Final Warning Before You Enter the Arena:
You don't need to be perfect.
You need to be clear, controlled, and clinically credible under stress.
Part I will teach you the terrain.

After that, it's time to train for real.

—CHKZ
Because if you're going to speak, make it count.

CHAPTER 1 - The Stakes Are Higher Than Just a Pass

OET as a Performance Arena, Not Just a Test

Trainer Trigger: "What's the real cost of Band B?"

CHAPTER AIM

Reframe OET from a language test to a high-stakes clinical performance zone that demands precision, pressure-proof communication, and professional presence.

LEARNING OUTCOMES

By the end of this chapter, candidates and trainers will be able to:

Demonstrate awareness of the clinical and career impact of OET results

Differentiate between passing and performing under pressure

Identify the hidden costs of underperformance (Band B)

Prioritise strategic preparation over passive practice

TACTICAL WARM-UP (Pressure Primer)

-- "Your visa, your licence, your future job — all depend on your next 2hours 45 minutes. Are you rehearsing like that's true?"

-- "A patient file lands on your desk. A consultant's watching. Your words decide what happens next. Ready?"

STRATEGIC ERROR

Thinking OET is 'just a test.'

Band C and Band B candidates often approach OET like it's a grammar quiz. They rehearse to pass, not to perform.

Result? Fluency collapses under pressure. Clinical clarity evaporates.

And Band A stays locked behind the door they didn't even realise they needed to open.

TACTICAL TRUTH

OET is not a test.

It's a rehearsal for trust.

You are not being tested on your English.

You are being assessed on whether a human being — under stress — can trust you with their care.

COMPONENT & CRITERIA BREAKDOWN

Test Part: All four OET sub-tests (L / R / W / S)

Criteria Tied:

Speaking: Clinical Communication, Fluency, Appropriateness

Writing: Genre, Conciseness, Relevance

Listening/Reading: Precision, Filtering, Relevance

Commentary:

Band A sounds like this:

"We'll run that test today. In the meantime, here's what you can expect."

Band B sounds like this:

"Er… maybe we will check it. You… maybe wait now, yes?"

Same message. Different outcome. One inspires calm. The other creates confusion.

MINDSET REFRAME: THE CLINICIAN'S UPGRADE

"Speak like a regulator's listening. Write like the referral will be read aloud."

You're not preparing for a mark. You're preparing for a moment when someone's safety depends on your sentence.

CHKZ STRATEGY INSTRUCTION

How to Train Like This is Real — Because It Is

CLINICIAN'S CHOICE

Stop asking: "What do I need to pass?"

Start asking:

– "What does the examiner need to hear to trust me?"

– "Would I follow these instructions if I were the patient?"

– "Can I explain this under pressure, without losing clinical control?"

PHRASES THAT WIN POINTS

– "Let me explain what will happen next…"

– "Just to clarify, are you currently experiencing…"

– "That's a very normal reaction. Here's what we'll do…"

EXAMINER TRIGGER POINT

When you hesitate, over-explain, or speak in circles — the examiner doesn't hear your English.

They hear: "This candidate will confuse real patients."

Every weak phrase costs trust. Every precise sentence earns it.

REAL-WORLD TRANSFER (CLINIC CROSSOVER)

This is not simulation.

In six months, that patient might be real.

That referral might land on an actual desk.

That phone call might be with someone's mother.

You're not training for test day.

You're rehearsing for every day that follows.

TRAINER NOTES & DIFFERENTIATION

Coaching Tip: Use video examples. Show what Band A looks like.

Assessor Watchpoint: Listen for risk-language — does the candidate hedge, delay, or deflect responsibility?

Peer Coaching Tip: Run **"Clinical Trust Challenges"** — where partners rate each other's clarity under stress.

Band B → Band A Mini-Rubric:

Skill	Band B (Functional)	Band A (Performance)
Speaking	Hesitant, vague, overly polite or unclear	Clear, concise, calm under pressure
Writing	Too much or too little information	Prioritised, purpose-driven, context-specific

TACTICAL APPLICATION ZONE (Blue-Diamond Drill)

Role-Play Challenge:

"You're explaining a delay in surgery to a family member. You have 90 seconds. Keep them calm and informed."

Decision Point Drill:

"What phrase would you not use — and why?"

Timed Phrase-Mapping:

Map 5 "safe" patient phrases to high-performance OET versions in under 2 minutes.

PERFORMANCE WRAP-UP (Chapter Plenary)

Aim Recap:

You're not here to pass. You're here to perform under pressure.

Clinician Coaching Recap:

– Trust is earned in your tone, clarity, and calm.

– Band A is built in your mouth, not just your memory.

– Train like your licence depends on it — because it might.

Self-Coaching Questions

"Did I speak like someone is relying on me?"

"Would I trust me, based on what I just said?"

"Am I performing, or just producing language?"

Trainer Challenge

Design a micro-scenario where a weak phrase creates a safety risk.

Have learners identify it, upgrade it, and defend their choice.

REFLECTION CHECKPOINT

"Is my communication calm — or just correct?"

"If I saw a Band B candidate in clinic, what would I worry about?"

"Would I pass me if the patient was my own child?"

CHAPTER 2 - Decoding the OET Battlefield

Sub-Test Breakdown, Scoring Mechanics, and Test-Day Psychology

Includes: Visual OET Command Map + Time-Pressure Matrix

CHAPTER AIM

Strip away test-day confusion. Arm candidates with clinical-level clarity across all four sub-tests — and show them how to execute under fire.

LEARNING OUTCOMES

By the end of this chapter, candidates and trainers will be able to:

Break down each OET sub-test into functional performance zones

Interpret official scoring rubrics and apply them tactically

Execute time-management strategies for each test component

Manage clinical mindset under exam pressure

TACTICAL WARM-UP (Pressure Primer)

– "You've got 5 minutes left and two questions unfinished. What do you drop — and why?"

– "Your pen slips mid-referral. Do you fix the grammar, or push forward with clarity?"

STRATEGIC ERROR

Approaching the test like a school exam.

Band C candidates try to 'finish every task' like it's a worksheet. They chase perfection and collapse under time.

Band B candidates often understand the tasks — but not the mechanics of how to score.

The real threat? Losing marks not from language failure… but from strategy blindness.

TACTICAL TRUTH

You're not just being tested on what you know — but on how well you deploy it under time, stress, and silence.

That makes this not an exam.

It makes it a performance pressure lab.

And you're the subject.

COMPONENT & CRITERIA BREAKDOWN

Test Parts:

Listening (A, B, C)

Reading (A, B, C)

Writing (profession-specific)

Speaking (2 role-plays)

Scoring Focus:

Each sub-test measures different performance indicators:

Sub-Test	Core Focus	Pressure Trap	Band A Response
Listening A	Note accuracy + clinical filtering	Writing everything or nothing	Filters essential facts, ignores filler
Reading B	Professional understanding	Panicking on unknown terms	Uses logic, context, and test literacy

Sub-Test	Core Focus	Pressure Trap	Band A Response
Writing	Genre, relevance, tone	Data dump or vague filler	Prioritises clinical need + conciseness
Speaking	Fluency, appropriateness, empathy	Robotic answers or emotional collapse	Clinically calm, patient-centred, efficient

VISUAL OET COMMAND MAP
(Insert stylised visual)
Breakdown showing:
Which mental muscles each sub-test demands
Where candidates typically choke under pressure
What success sounds and feels like under time constraints

TIME-PRESSURE MATRIX
OET isn't about finishing everything. It's about finishing what matters.

Train learners to:
Identify 'Must Win' zones in each test (e.g. Case Notes filtering, Part A listening keywords)
Know when to abandon, push forward, or slow down

Build 3-tier mental timers for:
Setup time
Execution time
Backup/review time

Example:

Sub-Test	Total Time	Danger Zone	Band A Strategy
Writing	45 mins	25 min case-notes trap	5-min skim → 30-min draft → 10-min edit
Listening A	real-time	Missed initial detail	Predict, prime, paraphrase early
Speaking	5 mins prep / 5 mins role-play	Panic in first 60 secs	Anchor opening: clinical calm, signposting

MINDSET REFRAME: THE CLINICIAN'S UPGRADE
"This isn't a classroom. It's your first day at work — and someone's watching."

Every sub-test is a stand-in for a real clinical moment:
Can you filter what matters during a rushed consultation? (Listening)
Can you locate key policy text fast in an emergency? (Reading)
Can you write a safe, useful handover without fluff? (Writing)
Can you stay calm and strategic during a patient conversation? (Speaking)

CHKZ STRATEGY INSTRUCTION
Decoding Each Sub-Test Like a Clinical Task

CLINICIAN'S CHOICE
Instead of asking: "What's the format?" — ask:
"What would a real clinician do here?"
"What does the examiner want to hear or see?"

"How do I show Band A-level prioritisation — not just language?"

PHRASES THAT WIN POINTS
– **Writing**: "Given the patient's current symptoms and history, a follow-up may be advisable."
– **Speaking**: "Just to clarify, have you been experiencing this daily?"
– **Listening**: Learn to anticipate answers based on consultation flow.

EXAMINER TRIGGER POINT
If your structure, tone, or logic breaks down — the examiner thinks:
"This person might fail under pressure in real life."
Band A = pressure-proof professionalism.
Not perfect grammar.

REAL-WORLD TRANSFER (CLINIC CROSSOVER)
You're training not just for test day — but for shift day.
No nurse can ask Google for the drug name mid-ward round.
No doctor can guess what the referral says when the CT report arrives.
No paramedic gets a second chance at explaining next steps to a distressed patient.
Every OET task simulates a real demand. That's why the stakes are real.

TRAINER NOTES & DIFFERENTIATION
Scaffold the Battlefield: Create laminated battle maps for each sub-test with time breakdowns, key verbs, and danger zones.
Watchpoint: Over-preparation for Writing often causes under-preparation for Listening. Balance drills.
Peer Drill Tip: Set sub-test stations. Rotate every 15 minutes with tactical tasks at each.

Band B → A Mini-Rubric:

Performance Area	Band B	Band A
Timing	Rushes or stalls	Strategic pacing
Prioritisation	Lists all ideas equally	Highlights what matters most
Stress Response	Hesitant, reactive	Predictive, calm under fire

TACTICAL APPLICATION ZONE (Blue-Diamond Drill)
Timer Challenge:
Complete a Reading Part B task under 3 minutes. Debrief what slowed you down.
Decision Drill:
Which errors are worth correcting mid-role-play — and which should be ignored to maintain fluency?
Mock Command Map Build:
Build a whiteboard map of all four sub-tests with keywords: strategy, emotion, language type, role.

PERFORMANCE WRAP-UP (Chapter Plenary)
Aim Recap:
OET is a test of strategy under pressure, not just skill.

Clinician Coaching Recap:
– Know the battlefield before you fight.
– Score points by thinking like a working clinician.
– Time is your asset or your assassin. Train it.

Self-Coaching Questions
"Where do I lose control under time?"
"Can I explain the goal of each sub-test in one sentence?"
"Am I training my thinking — or just my language?"

Trainer Challenge
Have your learners narrate their test-day plan aloud.
If it sounds like survival, reframe it to strategy.

REFLECTION CHECKPOINT
– "Am I preparing to pass, or preparing to perform?"
– "Would my test-day mindset work during a night shift?"
– "Do I react — or do I rehearse like a clinician?"

Up next:
Chapter 3 – The 12 Professions, One Standard
Because no matter your badge, Band A doesn't bend. Let's decode what's shared — and what's unique.

CHAPTER 3 - The 12 Professions, One Standard

What's Universal. What's Unique.

Includes: Profession Icons + QR-linked Bonus Vault Entries

CHAPTER AIM
Establish a unified standard for clinical performance communication while identifying the critical tweaks and nuances per profession.

LEARNING OUTCOMES
By the end of this chapter, candidates and trainers will be able to:
Identify the universal OET communication and assessment standards across all 12 professions
Differentiate the key task styles, expectations, and language registers by profession
Apply profession-specific strategies without losing sight of Band A benchmarks
Integrate shared success principles into customised training plans

TACTICAL WARM-UP (Pressure Primer)
– "You're a dietitian. A nurse. A vet. Does Band A care?"
– "You're in front of the examiner. Does your job title justify a communication breakdown?"

STRATEGIC ERROR
Assuming 'My profession is different, so the rules are different.'
Wrong.
The patient doesn't care if you're a speech pathologist or a pharmacist.
They care if they understand you, trust you, and feel safe.
OET is built on this principle. Band A doesn't flex for familiarity.

TACTICAL TRUTH
OET has one exam. One standard. One expectation: clinical communication under pressure.
Yes, the scenarios shift. The cases vary.
But the language? The professionalism? The empathy?
That's universal.

COMPONENT & CRITERIA BREAKDOWN
What's Shared Across All Professions?

OET uses a uniform scoring framework for:
Speaking
Writing

Core criteria across both:

Scoring Pillar	Applies to All 12 Professions
Clinical appropriateness	
Clarity and conciseness	
Tone and empathy	
Genre and register	
Organisation	

What Changes?

Scenario context

Profession-specific tasks

Case note complexity and terminology

Patient/Client interaction types

Functional language emphasis (e.g. instruction vs reassurance)

MINDSET REFRAME: THE CLINICIAN'S UPGRADE

"Your job title may change. But your communication standard never does."

Whether you're a physiotherapist adjusting posture or a dentist explaining extraction — your clarity, empathy, and control must hit the same professional ceiling.

Band A = clinically credible, linguistically precise, emotionally attuned. No exceptions.

STRATEGY SECTION – CHKZ TACTICAL INSTRUCTION

CLINICIAN'S CHOICE

For every profession, ask:

What kind of patient or client do I typically serve?

What type of information do I usually give or receive?

What is the worst outcome if I fail to communicate clearly?

Then train:

Functional chunks (e.g. "Let me show you how…" / "You might experience…")

Controlled tone shifts (calming vs instructive vs directive)

Register control (professional, not robotic)

PROFESSION SNAPSHOT GRID

Profession	Primary Communication Task	Danger Zone	Tactical Focus
Medicine	Diagnosis + referral	Over-explaining symptoms	Prioritise + transfer key info fast
Nursing	Monitoring + care instructions	Vague timelines or unclear tasks	Clarify frequency + next steps
Dentistry	Procedure prep + reassurance	Jargon overload	Rephrase technical terms
Pharmacy	Explaining dosage + contraindications	Robotic delivery of risks	Use patient-friendly warnings
Speech Pathology	Behavioural + progress explanation	Losing the family in technicality	Build rapport + check understanding
Physiotherapy	Guiding physical instructions	Fast or unclear commands	Clear, paced, stepwise directions
Audiology	Device explanation + hearing tests	Overloading with numbers	Simplify + visualise info
Radiography	Positioning + procedural clarity	Weak consent language	Calm directive tone + safety steps
Dietetics	Meal plans + behavioural adjustment	Over-explaining science	Link info to outcomes + habits

Profession	Primary Communication Task	Danger Zone	Tactical Focus
Occupational Therapy	Function-focused + family liaison	Overusing vague goals ("independence")	Concrete next steps
Veterinary	Owner reassurance + care instruction	Ignoring owner's emotion	Balance fact with empathy
Optometry	Vision tests + prescription advice	Clinical tone too detached	Conversational clarity

[**QR**: Access Bonus Profession Vault with sample role-plays + case notes per profession]

CHKZ TOOLS & PHRASES THAT WIN POINTS
Universal Phrases (All Professions):
– "Let me explain that another way…"
– "Would it help if I showed you how?"
– "Before we finish, can I just check you're clear on…"
– "Some people feel worried at this point — that's completely normal."

Profession-Specific Adaptations (Examples):
Pharmacy: "This medicine may cause drowsiness — so avoid driving after taking it."
Veterinary: "It's common for dogs to limp slightly after this injection — it should settle within 24 hours."
Radiography: "You'll hear a loud clicking noise, but it's completely normal — just try to remain still."

REAL-WORLD TRANSFER (CLINIC CROSSOVER)
Healthcare professionals don't switch off their communication skills by badge.
Patients don't care that you're "just" a pharmacist — they want answers, clarity, and safety.
Pet owners won't tolerate dismissiveness from a vet — they need reassurance and trust.
Radiographers and audiologists deal with real fear — not just positioning.
Professional credibility = communication credibility.
Train for the standard, not the title.

TRAINER NOTES & DIFFERENTIATION
Coach Per Profession: Highlight top 5 common errors for each role (vocab, tone, logic gaps)
Visual Wall: Use icons per profession across resources to reinforce identity + standard alignment
Peer Teaching Tip: Let candidates from different professions cross-teach sample scripts

Band B → Band A Rubric Add-on:
Focus	Band B	Band A
Role Clarity	Profession comes through eventually	Clear tone, scope, and patient framing
Empathy Language	Generic or vague phrases	Contextualised, calm, emotionally tuned
Clinical Logic	Slightly muddled flow	Sequential, safety-prioritised delivery

TACTICAL APPLICATION ZONE (Blue-Diamond Drill)
30-sec Flash Role-play: Pick your profession. You've got 30 seconds to explain a standard procedure to a nervous client. Go.
Sentence Rewrite Challenge: Take a cold, technical sentence. Reframe it for patient clarity and warmth.
Compare & Reflect: Vet explains post-op care vs Nurse explains discharge steps — what sounds the same? What must change?

PERFORMANCE WRAP-UP (Chapter Plenary)
Aim Recap:
<u>Profession-specific prep is smart. But the standard stays high, no matter your badge.</u>

Clinician Coaching Recap:
– One exam. One level. One patient experience.
– Customise your vocabulary — not your professionalism.
– Empathy is not optional. It's clinical currency.

Self-Coaching Questions
"Have I trained for my profession — or hidden behind it?"
"Would I pass if they swapped my role cards today?"
"Do I sound like a safe, respected professional — regardless of the label?"

Trainer Challenge
<u>Run a "Badge Swap Drill":</u>
Have students perform role-plays in a different profession — then debrief what changed, and what didn't.

REFLECTION CHECKPOINT
– "Would I trust me — based on how I speak?"
– "Am I prioritising clarity and care — or just completing the script?"
– "What part of my role must shine in my communication?"

Next up: Chapter 4 – Textbook English vs Tactical English
Because your grammar book won't save you when the Patient panics or the clock runs out. Let's sharpen the language that actually wins the grade — and the moment.

CHAPTER 4 - Textbook English vs Tactical English

What Band A Sounds Like Under Pressure

Includes: Examiner Red Flag Callouts – Weak Language Traps to Kill Now

CHAPTER AIM

To expose the fatal gap between academic English and tactical clinical communication — and upgrade your language to Band A performance under pressure.

LEARNING OUTCOMES

By the end of this chapter, candidates and trainers will be able to:

Identify common Band C expressions that fail under clinical pressure

Replace textbook phrases with Band A clinical alternatives

Demonstrate strategic tone, structure, and function under test-time constraints

Adapt language on the spot to suit patient needs, clinical tasks, and time limits

TACTICAL WARM-UP (Pressure Primer)

– "The patient just fainted. You say, 'He became unconscious.' Examiner says… Band B."

– "Your role-play timer hits 2 minutes left. You're still explaining basic symptoms. What now?"

STRATEGIC ERROR

Thinking 'good grammar' equals Band A.

Wrong battlefield.

Textbook English may be grammatically clean —

But it often lacks:

Clinical tone

Contextual relevance

Emotional calibration

Time-sensitive precision

That's what costs you Band A.

TACTICAL TRUTH

OET isn't testing how many words you know. It's testing which ones you choose — under fire.

Band A = fluent, focused, professional.

You don't just speak correctly.

You speak like it matters.

COMPONENT & CRITERIA BREAKDOWN

Sub-Test. Speaking

Relevant Criteria:

Appropriateness of Language

Clarity of Expression

Fluency

Clinical Communication Effectiveness

What Band A Sounds Like Under Pressure:

Band C (Textbook)	Band A (Tactical)
"You will take this tablet two times."	"Take one tablet in the morning and one at night."
"Don't worry, it's okay."	"It's normal to feel anxious — let me explain what happens next."
"The patient had high temperature."	"You've had a fever — that could explain the tiredness."
"I suggest that you should…"	"One option is to…" or "We could consider…"
"Please try to avoid to smoke."	"It's important to cut down smoking — even small changes help."

MINDSET REFRAME: THE CLINICIAN'S UPGRADE
"You're not a walking dictionary. You're a clinical communicator under pressure."

Every word must:
Build trust
Convey care
Clarify clinical info
Move the consultation forward
If it doesn't? Cut it.

STRATEGY SECTION – CHKZ TACTICAL INSTRUCTION

CLINICIAN'S CHOICE
Switch from narration to action.

Examples:
"Your blood pressure is high." → "We need to bring it down to reduce risk."
"You may take this medicine." → "Start with one tablet — I'll show you when to take it."
Band A language = ownership + outcome.

PHRASES THAT WIN POINTS

To Show Empathy:
– "That must be uncomfortable — let's talk through how we'll manage it."
– "It's completely understandable to feel that way."
– "Many people feel worried — you're not alone."

To Give Clear Instructions:
– "Take this with food to avoid stomach upset."
– "Try this for the next three days — if there's no improvement, come back."
– "Let's check one more thing before you leave."

To Reassure Professionally:
– "It sounds worrying, but the symptoms you've described are common and treatable."
– "We've seen this before — you're in safe hands."
– "There are clear next steps we can take."

To Show Shared Decision-Making:
– "Would you like me to explain the options again?"

– "We can go through the side effects together, if that helps."
– "What concerns you most about this treatment?"

EXAMINER TRIGGER POINT
Language Red Flags That Drop Your Score:
Repeating textbook memorised phrases
Empty reassurances (e.g. "Don't worry")
Over-politeness without clarity
Jargon without explanation
Describing symptoms instead of managing them

REAL-WORLD TRANSFER (CLINIC CROSSOVER)
Textbook English might pass an academic test.
It won't build trust with a real patient.

Tactical English is the difference between:
– Confusion vs Confidence
– Liability vs Leadership
– Recitation vs Rapport
In real practice, patients don't want a grammar lesson. They want clarity, comfort, and a safe hand to follow.

TRAINER NOTES & DIFFERENTIATION
Coach Band C → Band A rewrites in every role-play
Run "SAY IT BETTER" drills: swap dull textbook phrases for tactical ones
Highlight clinical verbs: monitor, manage, assess, reassure, reduce, refer

Peer Coaching Tip: Give learners a red pen and let them mark each other's weak phrases live

Weak Phrase Type	Trainer Correction Strategy
Over-formality	Rephrase with natural tone
Robotic structures	Add empathy + action
Confusing sequences	Restructure for clinical flow
Empty filler phrases	Replace with outcome-focused lines

TACTICAL APPLICATION ZONE (Blue-Diamond Drill)
Sentence Surgery Drill
Take these Band C lines and rewrite them for clarity + clinical impact:
"The patient has a pain in his chest."
"Please wait for five minutes before go home."
"I advise you don't eat sugar."

30-Second Upgrade Challenge
You've got 30 seconds:
– Reassure an anxious patient using Band A empathy
– Explain a medication routine in plain English
– Correct a patient's misunderstanding — without blame

Decision Point Flashcards
Choose:

– "Say it like a textbook"
– "Say it like a clinician under pressure"
Use cards to test responses under time constraints.

PERFORMANCE WRAP-UP (Chapter Plenary)
CHAPTER MISSION Recap:
Tactical English is precise, professional, and pressure-proof.

Clinician Coaching Recap:
– Speak like someone will quote you in court.
– Don't explain symptoms. Manage them.
– Rehearse clarity — not perfection.

3 Self-Coaching Questions
"Did I sound like a clinician — or a textbook?"
"Would a patient feel safe hearing me explain that?"
"What phrase did I improve most this week?"

Trainer Challenge
Record 2 versions of a candidate's response:
– Textbook-style
– Tactical Band A version
Then play both back and debrief: Which one earns trust? Which one earns points?

REFLECTION CHECKPOINT
– "Do I control my words — or just release them?"
– "Would I trust this advice if I were the patient?"
– "What phrase in my clinical vocabulary must be deleted today?"

Next Up: PART 2 – THE SKILLS
We move from battlefield mindset to sharp communication moves.
From strategy to skill.
Because you don't just know how to pass — you need to perform like you've already earned it.

PART I WRAP-UP

REFLECT. RESET. REFOCUS.

Know the Game. Play to Win.

Tactical Debrief
Let's be brutally clear.
You're not preparing for a test.
You're preparing for performance under time, pressure, and scrutiny — with patient trust, clinical credibility, and career trajectory on the line.

Part I: The Arena trained your eye on what others miss:
The real cost of Band B isn't just a lower score — it's delayed visas, missed jobs, and crushed confidence.
The OET is not just a test of language — it's a battlefield of decisions, framed by psychology, criteria, and time.
Each of the 12 healthcare professions carries different case types — but shares the same bar of clarity, care, and control.

Textbook English? It survives in theory.
Tactical English? It survives in triage.
This isn't about sounding clever.
It's about sounding clinically competent — and proving it under pressure.

Core Shifts So Far

From	To
"Learn English"	"Deliver clinical communication"
"Hope I pass"	"Train like I must perform"
"Just follow the sample"	"Read the room, lead the moment"
"Any Band will do"	"Only Band A protects my future"

Reset Your Intentions
Before you step into the next chapters, ask yourself:
Am I training like someone whose future depends on this?
Have I studied the rules of the arena — or am I still winging it?
Am I still using phrases that sound safe... but score low?

What Comes Next
Part II shifts the spotlight to skill mastery: Listening. Reading. Writing. Speaking.
You'll get:
Precision tools
High-band tactics
Scoring logic from an examiner's lens
Real-time pressure strategies
This is where preparation becomes performance-proof.

3 Reflection Prompts

Write these down. Don't skip.

These are your internal training reps — and they matter more than you think.

"What must I now stop doing — immediately — if I'm serious about reaching Band A?"

"Which lesson from these first chapters hit hardest — and how will I apply it this week?"

"What would it look like if I trained like a clinical professional, not just a test candidate?"

Part I is complete. The gloves are off. The game is real.

Now let's sharpen your skills — and raise your score.

Onward to Part II – THE SKILLS: Sharpen What Scores. Perform What Matters.

PART 2 – SPEAK TO LEAD

OET Speaking Mastery Under Pressure

The Test Is Speaking.
The Real Test Is Leadership Under Fire.

Let's be clear.

The OET Speaking test isn't just about pronunciation, politeness, or remembering a script.
It's about professional presence — under artificial time limits, unnatural prompts, and invisible scoring pressure.
It's about walking into a mock consultation… and showing you could lead a real one tomorrow.

Band A isn't just about sounding fluent.

It's about sounding like someone who belongs in the room.
Who patients trust.
Who juniors watch.
Who speaks with clinical clarity and human control — even when the patient is panicked, the scenario is messy, and time is ticking.

What This Part Covers — And Why It Matters

Chapter 5 – Command the Conversation
Clinical tone, empathy control, non-verbal command
You'll learn how to lead the dialogue like a professional — not just speak like a candidate.
Vault Bonus: Voice of Authority Drill — retrain how you sound under pressure.

Chapter 6 – The Speaking Criteria Unlocked
What each score point really means in practice
No more guessing what "appropriateness" or "linguistic resources" actually mean.
Includes: Band B vs A comparison clips with commentary.

Chapter 7 – High-Stakes Language That Lands
Phrase banks, transitions, recovery lines
Build your Band A vocabulary — not just for fluency, but for command.
Uses: phrases that win points tactical format.

Chapter 8 Role-Plays for All 12 Professions
Prompt + model + commentary x12
Each profession. Every pressure type. With trainer notes and rubrics to sharpen delivery.
Includes: CEFR–OET mapping and self-scoring tools.

Strategic Warning
Here's what weak candidates do:
Memorise scripts and freeze when the role-play shifts
Smile politely but lose control of the conversation
Apologise instead of redirecting

Speak fluently but without clinical focus or empathy calibration

Here's what Band A performers do:
Speak with the patient, not at them
Prioritise clinical tasks and time management
Use tone as a leadership tool
Adapt the conversation, own the moment, finish strong

Why This Part Matters
Because leadership happens through language.
And in the Speaking test, you either take the lead — or you follow the prompt into mediocrity.

This section will train your:
Tone control (because kindness without clarity isn't safe)
Phrase command (because vague language doesn't win points)
Pressure handling (because nerves kill Band A when left unchecked)
Real-time decision making (because the test doesn't pause for perfection)

Final Prep Thought
This isn't a speaking test.
It's a clinical leadership simulation.
You're not just scored on words.
You're scored on how you guide, explain, reassure, and respond in real time.
If Part 1 taught you the game...
Part 2 turns you into a player who can win it — sentence by sentence.
Let's raise your voice.
And your value.

Next: Chapter 5 – Command the Conversation: Clinical Tone, Empathy Control, Non-Verbal Authority

CHAPTER 5 – COMMAND THE CONVERSATION

Clinical Tone. Empathy Control. Non-Verbal Command.

Vault Add-On: Voice of Authority Drill

CHAPTER MISSION
Train candidates to speak with clinical control, tone authority, and calm empathy under performance pressure.

LEARNING OUTCOMES
By the end of this chapter, you will:
Deliver clinical information with tonal authority and clarity
Demonstrate empathy without weakening leadership
Control non-verbal signals that project confidence and command
Adapt your vocal delivery to match patient distress or concern
Respond to pressure without emotional leakage

TACTICAL WARM-UP (PRESSURE PRIMER)
A patient interrupts you mid-explanation and demands faster answers. How do you respond without losing control?
You need to correct the patient's dangerous self-diagnosis — without sounding arrogant or dismissive. What tone wins trust?

STRATEGIC ERROR
Friendly but weak.
Candidates who aim for "warmth" often end up sounding vague, passive, or too soft.

This leads to:
Under-explaining risks
Letting the patient dominate the structure
Sounding unsure or hesitant when reassurance is needed

TACTICAL TRUTH
Empathy without clarity is unsafe.
Leadership tone means sounding calm, in control, and grounded — even while being kind.
You are not just being assessed on what you say.
You are being judged on how you own the moment.

COMPONENT & CRITERIA BREAKDOWN
OET Speaking Sub-Test

Relevant Criteria:
Appropriateness of Language
Clarity of Speech
Relationship-building
Fluency and Tone Control

What Band A sounds like under pressure:
"I understand your concern. Let me explain what this means for your next steps."
[**Tone**: measured, composed, professional — without robotic detachment.]

MINDSET REFRAME: THE CLINICIAN'S UPGRADE

Speak like a team will act on your words.

If a nurse takes your instruction or a patient acts on your advice — is your tone clear, credible, and decisive enough?

CHKZ TACTICAL INSTRUCTION

CLINICIAN'S CHOICE: MASTERING YOUR TONE

Tone tools:

Slow initial sentence = authority

Mid-volume + downward intonation = control

Brief pauses = reflection and command

Test-pressure upgrade:

If you feel nerves rising — drop your pitch, slow your pace, and breathe before responding.

Train yourself to default to control, not panic.

PHRASES THAT WIN POINTS

Situation	Tactical Phrase
Reassuring without overpromising	"It's understandable to feel that way — here's what we can do now."
Calming a worried patient	"Let's take this one step at a time together."
Resetting the direction	"If I may, let's return to the main issue you mentioned earlier."
Setting professional boundaries	"I appreciate your input — here's the safest course of action I'd recommend."

EXAMINER TRIGGER POINT

Red Flag: High-speed, high-pitch speaking = stress.

Examiners will mark you down for rushed, breathless delivery — even if the words are correct.

Band A candidates control their vocal speed and presence.

PROFESSION EXAMPLES

Radiographer: "I'll talk you through the steps before we begin the procedure." (Low-pitch, guiding tone)

Pharmacist: "This medication must be taken exactly as prescribed — here's how." (Assertive, reassuring)

Physiotherapist: "You may feel discomfort, but I'll explain how to manage that safely." (Empathetic without collapse)

CLINIC CROSSOVER

In real practice, tone builds or breaks trust.

A rushed or apologetic delivery in front of patients or team members damages your professional image.

Leadership starts with how you sound — not just what you know.

TRAINER NOTES & DIFFERENTIATION

Coach stronger candidates to fine-tune delivery pace and pause placement

For lower levels, focus on repeating high-impact phrases with accurate tone

Peer Coaching Tip: Use phone recording + playback with tone checklist

Mini-Rubric:

Band B: Polite, mostly clear, slight pitch shifts or speed issues

Band A: Calm, anchored, authoritative delivery with adaptive tone shifts

BLUE-DIAMOND DRILL (TACTICAL APPLICATION ZONE)
30-Second Delivery Challenge
→ **Scenario**: You're explaining a delayed test result to a concerned patient.
Record yourself. Play it back. Would you trust this voice?

Role-Play Upgrade
→ Take a standard script. Rewrite it using phrases that win points. Now re-perform it with controlled tone.

PERFORMANCE WRAP-UP (CHAPTER PLENARY)
You are the voice they trust. Or the one they forget.
Tone = Leadership.
Presence = Authority.
This chapter trained you to lead with your voice — not just fill silence with speech.

3 Self-Coaching Questions:
"Did I speak with command — or just with words?"
"Would a real patient feel safer after hearing me?"
"Did I control my tone — or did it control me?"

Trainer Challenge:
Replay a Band A recording. Transcribe the phrases and note the tone features.
Then coach a partner to replicate them — under timed pressure.

Next: Chapter 6 – The Speaking Criteria Unlocked
What each score point really means in practice — with annotated samples and scoring clarity.

CHAPTER 6 – THE SPEAKING CRITERIA UNLOCKED

What Each Score Point Really Means in Practice

Bonus: Annotated Band B vs A Comparison Clips (QR-linked)

CHAPTER MISSION
Turn the OET speaking criteria from vague labels into concrete, coachable performance behaviours under test pressure.

LEARNING OUTCOMES
By the end of this chapter, you will:
Interpret each OET Speaking criterion in Band A–B performance terms
Differentiate between "good enough" and "clinically excellent" speaking
Apply self-assessment tools using Band A-level behaviours
Spot Band B red flags and upgrade them in real time
Coach peer and self-performance with precision

TACTICAL WARM-UP (PRESSURE PRIMER)
You think you did "well" in your last role-play — but can you explain why?
If the examiner asked: "What was weak about your fluency today?", would you have an answer?

STRATEGIC ERROR
Learning the labels. Not the behaviours.

Most candidates memorise the criteria names: intelligibility, appropriateness, etc.
But they never translate those into tactical, observable actions.

TACTICAL TRUTH
Band A isn't a mystery. It's a method.
The difference between Band B and Band A is not intelligence or kindness.
It's consistency, clarity, command, and control under timed pressure.

COMPONENT & CRITERIA BREAKDOWN
OET Speaking – Performance Descriptors

There are 9 official scoring dimensions, grouped into two categories:
Linguistic Criteria
Intelligibility
Fluency
Appropriateness of Language
Resources of Grammar and Expression

Clinical Communication Criteria
Relationship-building
Understanding and Incorporating the Patient's Perspective
Providing Structure
Information-giving
Listening and Responding

MINDSET REFRAME: THE CLINICIAN'S UPGRADE

Don't think like a student. Think like a clinical performer.
The examiner isn't scoring your personality.
They're scoring your clarity, strategy, and safety under time constraints.

CHKZ TACTICAL INSTRUCTION

BAND B vs BAND A – THE REAL DIFFERENCE

CRITERION	BAND B	BAND A
Intelligibility	Mostly clear, some minor strain	Crystal-clear, minimal effort to understand
Fluency	Occasional hesitations or repair	Smooth, confident, strategically paced
Appropriateness	Generally suitable	Consistently adapted to tone, context, and hierarchy
Grammar/Expression	Good control, minor slips	Flexible, precise, wide range with no breakdown
Relationship-building	Friendly, supportive	Supportive and controlled; leader–patient dynamic clear
Understanding Patient	Reactively responsive	Proactively integrates patient concerns early
Structure	Mostly logical	Razor-sharp, signposted, zero derailment
Information-giving	Clear, but long or basic	Prioritised, chunked, clinically strategic
Listening/Responding	Engaged and reactive	Predictive, adaptive, responsive with direction

BAND COMPARISON CLIP ANALYSIS (VAULT ADD-ON)
Use the QR-linked vault to:
Hear real Band B vs A responses

Use the CHKZ Analysis Strip to mark:
Fillers
Weak tone
Lost structure
Strong repair
Command transitions
Then coach up.

EXAMINER RED FLAGS

No signposting: "Okay... so..." instead of "Let me walk you through…"
Vague empathy: "Don't worry, it's fine" instead of "It's understandable to feel that way. Here's what I'd suggest."
Over-explaining: Drowning in detail without prioritisation
Weak close: "I think that's all" vs "Just to summarise, your next steps are…"

PHRASES THAT SCORE HIGH

CRITERION	HIGH-SCORING PHRASE
Structure	"First, I'll explain what we've found. Then I'll walk you through the next steps."
Empathy	"You've raised an important concern, and I want to address that clearly."
Clarity	"In simple terms, this means your blood pressure is above the safe range."
Closing	"Let's check your understanding before we wrap up."

PROFESSION EXAMPLES

Optometrist: "Before we proceed, let me outline what each test is for — so you feel confident."

Speech Pathologist: "I've noted the hesitation — let's use a simple repetition task next."

Dietitian: "You mentioned struggling with appetite — would you be open to adjusting meal timing first?"

CLINIC CROSSOVER

In real healthcare:

A Band B communicator gets polite nods

A Band A communicator gets follow-through

They sound like the person in charge, even when they're kind.

That makes patients act, not just listen.

TRAINER NOTES & DIFFERENTIATION

For lower bands: Simplify the criteria to 3 words per score (e.g., "Clear–Fluent–Calm")

Use side-by-side audio playback to contrast performance

Peer Rubric: Use CHKZ strips during live mock role-plays

Band B → Band A Mini-Coaching Tip: "How would a senior nurse say that under pressure?"

BLUE-DIAMOND DRILL (TACTICAL APPLICATION ZONE)

30-Second Criteria Replay

Listen to your mock role-play. Choose one criterion (e.g. structure).

Write 2 things you did well + 1 upgrade to apply next time.

Sentence Rewrite

Original: "I think you should maybe take the medicine."

Band A Rewrite: "Based on your symptoms, I'd strongly recommend starting the medication today."

PERFORMANCE WRAP-UP (CHAPTER PLENARY)

You're not aiming for mystery marks.

You're building measurable behaviours.

Knowing the criteria is passive.

Scoring Band A is strategic.

3 Self-Coaching Questions:

"Which criterion is currently my weakest?"

"What does Band A performance sound like for my profession?"

"Can I explain my score — and defend it?"

Trainer Challenge:

Record a 3-minute sample. Score yourself blindly using the 9-point breakdown.

Now… swap it with a partner and compare. Did you judge fairly?

Next: Chapter 7 – High-Stakes Language That Lands

Phrase banks. Recovery lines. Tactical transitions. This is where you win or lose Band A.

CHAPTER 7 – HIGH-STAKES LANGUAGE THAT LANDS

Phrase Banks, Transitions, Recovery Lines That Win Under Fire

PHRASES THAT WIN POINTS FORMAT

CHAPTER MISSION
Arm yourself with Band A clinical language — under pressure, in real time, without sounding robotic.

LEARNING OUTCOMES
By the end of this chapter, you will:
Deploy high-impact phrases for clarity, control, and compassion
Recover from errors or tension with professional redirection language
Use tactical transitions to maintain structure and pace
Filter textbook English into usable, high-stakes chunks
Build a personal phrase bank that scores — and transfers to clinic life

TACTICAL WARM-UP (PRESSURE PRIMER)
A Patient just challenged your advice — what do you say next?
You forgot a word mid-sentence — how do you recover like a pro?

STRATEGIC ERROR
Winging it with good intentions.

Under pressure, most candidates default to vague, friendly English:
"Don't worry, everything will be okay."
"It's not that bad."
"I think maybe this is good for you."
That's not Band A. That's Band Unprepared.

TACTICAL TRUTH
Band A doesn't mean fancy. It means functional.
Scoring language is:
Precise
Professional
Pressure-proof
Purpose-driven

COMPONENT & CRITERIA BREAKDOWN
OET Speaking – Where Language Wins or Loses:

Appropriateness of Language: Is this the tone a clinician would use?
Grammar & Expression: Is it accurate, flexible, and fluent?
Information Giving: Are you chunking, signposting, and checking understanding?
Listening & Responding: Can you pivot, rephrase, or recover?

MINDSET REFRAME: THE CLINICIAN'S UPGRADE

You're not "talking to a Patient."
You're guiding a conversation in a clinical setting — with legal, emotional, and ethical consequences.
Your words carry weight. Use them like a professional.

PHRASES THAT WIN POINTS – CATEGORISED FOR COMBAT

1. OPENING THE INTERACTION

FUNCTION	PHRASE
Welcome	"Good morning, I'm Dr [Name] — I'll be taking care of you today."
Rapport	"I understand you've had quite a morning — let's get things sorted."
Clarifying purpose	"Just so I'm clear — you're here today about the discomfort in your chest, is that right?"

2. TRANSITIONING BETWEEN STAGES

FUNCTION	PHRASE
Moving to history	"Let me ask a few background questions first, just to build the full picture."
Explaining next step	"Next, I'd like to discuss the results we received — is that okay?"
Structuring delivery	"I'll break this down into three short parts: the issue, the options, and the plan."

3. EXPLAINING CLEARLY & SIMPLY

FUNCTION	PHRASE
Defining terms	"To put it simply, this means your blood pressure is consistently higher than safe levels."
Simplifying	"This infection is common — it just means your body is fighting off some bacteria."
Framing importance	"It's not urgent, but it is important — and needs attention soon."

4. RECOVERING FROM MISTAKES OR UNCERTAINTY

FUNCTION	PHRASE
Self-correction	"Let me rephrase that more clearly…"
Forgetting a term	"The word escapes me for a second — but let me explain it another way."
Resetting flow	"Let's go back a step so I can explain that properly."

5. SHOWING EMPATHY WITHOUT SOUNDING WEAK

FUNCTION	PHRASE
Validating concerns	"It's completely understandable to feel worried when symptoms don't improve."
Professional reassurance	"I've reviewed your case carefully, and I want you to know there's a clear path forward."
Anchoring empathy in action	"We'll take this one step at a time — and I'll guide you through each stage."

6. CHECKING UNDERSTANDING & INVITING CLARIFICATION

FUNCTION	PHRASE
Understanding	"Does that explanation make sense so far?"
Encouraging questions	"Before we move on — is there anything you'd like me to go over again?"

FUNCTION	PHRASE
Confirming message	"Could you repeat back the key steps — just so we're on the same page?"

7. DEALING WITH CHALLENGING INTERACTIONS

FUNCTION	PHRASE
De-escalation	"Let's slow down for a second — I want to make sure I've understood you fully."
Anchoring control	"I hear your concern — and I'm going to address it step by step."
Reframing	"Rather than focusing on the delay, let's look at what we can act on now."

8. CLOSING THE ROLE-PLAY STRONGLY

FUNCTION	PHRASE
Action recap	"So just to summarise: we'll start the new medication, monitor your response, and check in next week."
Confidence close	"You're doing the right thing by seeking help — and we'll tackle this together."
Parting phrase	"Thanks for your time today — and if anything feels off, don't hesitate to reach out."

CLINICIAN'S CHOICE – ADAPT BY PROFESSION

Radiographer: "You might hear some loud clicks — that's normal. The machine is just capturing detailed images."

Physiotherapist: "Let's go at your pace — and if something feels uncomfortable, just let me know immediately."

Pharmacist: "This tablet should be taken with food to avoid stomach irritation. Any questions before I go over side effects?"

REAL-WORLD TRANSFER (CLINIC CROSSOVER)

The same language that gets Band A is the language that builds trust in real hospitals.

This is not "test language." This is leadership language.

Patients remember how you made them feel.

Staff remember if you were clear or confusing.

You remember if you led the moment — or lost it.

TRAINER NOTES & DIFFERENTIATION

Beginner: Introduce 5 core phrases from each function area

Intermediate: Swap basic textbook language with targeted tactical upgrades

Advanced: Drill phrases under time pressure + role-specific cues

Peer Task: Pair students. One speaks, one ticks off "phrases that land"

Band B → Band A Mini-Rubric

Marker	Band B	Band A
Transitions	"Okay…"	"Now let's move to…"
Empathy	"Don't worry"	"It's understandable — here's our next step."
Recovery	Silence or "Umm…"	"Let me rephrase that more clearly…"

BLUE-DIAMOND DRILLS (TACTICAL APPLICATION ZONE)

Decision-Point Upgrade

Original: "You must exercise more."

Upgrade: "To support your recovery, I'd recommend light daily walks — how does that sound?"

Role-Play: Tactical Insertion Challenge

Partner A delivers a role-play. Partner B must insert at least:

One transition phrase

One recovery phrase

One empathy anchor

Score each for fluency, natural tone, and appropriateness.

PERFORMANCE WRAP-UP (CHAPTER PLENARY)

You don't win Band A with filler.

You win it with functional fluency and strategic speech.

3 Self-Coaching Prompts:

"Which of today's phrases do I already use confidently?"

"Which areas (transitions, recovery, empathy) are missing from my real speech?"

"Can I speak like a clinician before I become one?"

Trainer Challenge:

Take a 60-second video of a mock consultation.

Play it back. Count how many Band A phrases were used.

Then… upgrade one phrase in every category.

Next: Chapter 8 – Role-Plays for All 12 Professions

No more generic practice. This is the arena — with mapped scoring, model answers, and full-spectrum pressure.

CHAPTER 8 - Role-Plays for All 12 Professions

Prompt + Model + Commentary x12

Now with Trainer Strip, CEFR–OET Mapping, + Self-Scoring Rubric

CHAPTER AIM

Equip candidates from all 12 professions to rehearse, score, and upgrade their role-play performance under real test pressure.

LEARNING OUTCOMES

By the end of this chapter, candidates will be able to:

Demonstrate clinical communication aligned with their profession

Deliver structured responses under timed conditions

Apply Band A criteria to their own role-play performance

Identify tactical upgrades in tone, empathy, and recovery

Score themselves and peers using a clear rubric

TACTICAL WARM-UP (Pressure Primer)

"You've got two minutes to read the prompt. Your heart is racing. What do you plan first—tone, transitions, or timing?"

"A Patient just snapped at you mid-roleplay. What language stabilises the moment while keeping clinical control?"

STRATEGIC ERROR

Generic Tone, Over-Rehearsed Answers

Candidates default to memorised phrases or unnatural 'textbook' English, causing examiner disengagement and clinical credibility loss. Band C responses often sound robotic, hesitant, or overly formulaic.

TACTICAL TRUTH

Own the Prompt. Command the Role. Connect Like a Clinician.

Real Band A communication sounds spontaneous, safe, and strategic—layered with clinical calm, empathy control, and natural phrase upgrades. The role-play isn't a test—it's a clinical simulation.

COMPONENT & CRITERIA BREAKDOWN

Sub-Test: Speaking

Relevant Criteria:

Clinical Communication Effectiveness

Appropriateness of Language

Relationship Building

Information Gathering + Delivery

Intelligibility (Pronunciation, Fluency, Tone)

What Band A Sounds Like Under Pressure

Responds, doesn't react

Controls pace, tone, and recovery

Doesn't over-explain—filters by relevance

Anchors every phrase in clinical logic and empathy

MINDSET REFRAME: THE CLINICIAN'S UPGRADE

"You're not playing a role—you are the role."
Speak like a licensed professional, not a language candidate. Assume authority. Deliver clarity. Stay in charge—even when the patient panics, doubts, or disagrees.

CHKZ TACTICAL INSTRUCTION
Each of the 12 professions will include:
One full test-ready prompt
One Band A model response
One trainer commentary strip
CEFR–OET mapping breakdown
Self-scoring rubric aligned to test criteria

PROFESSIONAL ROLE-PLAY MODULES
MEDICINE
Prompt: Explain medication adjustment post-hospital discharge
Model: Concise, calming, clinically assertive
Focus: Polypharmacy + Patient safety concerns

NURSING
Prompt: Reassure a family member of a confused elderly patient
Model: Warmth with clinical authority
Focus: Repetition control + Safeguarding tone

PHYSIOTHERAPY
Prompt: Motivate a reluctant post-op patient
Model: Assertive, step-by-step coaching
Focus: Reframing pain + Compliance tone

DENTISTRY
Prompt: Explain extraction risks to an anxious patient
Model: Calm, non-patronising, precision tone
Focus: De-escalation phrases + clarity of consequence

PHARMACY
Prompt: Warn about antibiotic misuse
Model: Confident, informative, preventive
Focus: Legal vs advisory tone

VETERINARY
Prompt: Discuss post-surgical care for a pet
Model: Balance empathy with scientific delivery
Focus: Avoiding humanisation traps + clear owner instructions

OCCUPATIONAL THERAPY
Prompt: Support a patient returning home post-stroke
Model: Reassuring, forward-facing, structured
Focus: Goal setting + environmental control

SPEECH PATHOLOGY

Prompt: Reassure parent of child with speech delay
Model: Gentle, empowering, technical made simple
Focus: Normalisation vs over-promise

PODIATRY

Prompt: Explain diabetic foot care routine
Model: Precise, cautionary, routine-focused
Focus: Repetition + phrasing for habit formation

RADIOGRAPHY

Prompt: Prepare patient for MRI + contrast risks
Model: Calm, step-by-step, procedural clarity
Focus: Instructional tone + reaction management

DIETETICS

Prompt: Guide a patient post-bariatric surgery
Model: Clear, motivating, respectful of limits
Focus: Language of compliance + motivational tone

OPTOMETRY

Prompt: Discuss dry eye management with a patient
Model: Preventive, informative, professionally light
Focus: Ongoing management + lifestyle phrasing

REAL-WORLD TRANSFER (CLINIC CROSSOVER)

Every phrase, every prompt, every pause—mirrors the real world. These aren't just test drills. They're simulations of what real clinicians must deliver daily: structure, safety, and confidence under pressure.

TRAINER NOTES & DIFFERENTIATION

Pair low-confidence learners with stronger speakers using timed rounds
Use the Trainer Strip to model CEFR shifts (B2→C1 language upgrades)
Rubric can be colour-coded for peer feedback sessions
Watchpoints: excessive apologising, robotic phrasing, over-talking
Scoring Tip: Use the "Professional Presence" marker as a Band A decider

TACTICAL APPLICATION ZONE (BLUE-DIAMOND DRILL)
30-Second Roleplay Challenge:
Spin the Roleplay Wheel (QR-linked)
30 seconds to read, 90 seconds to respond
Score each other using the rubric

Role Rewind:
Play back a recorded role-play
Annotate: What worked? What weakened the message?

Phrase Reconstruction Drill:
Fix 3 Band C phrases
Upgrade them to Band A

PERFORMANCE WRAP-UP (CHAPTER PLENARY)

Aim Recap:

You don't pass the OET by guessing what to say. You pass by performing like a clinician. These 12 models are more than templates—they're mirrors, drills, and blueprints.

Self-Coaching Questions:

Which role-play challenged your tone or structure most?

What Band A phrase from another profession can you borrow for yours?

How will you train recovery lines and time-pressure control this week?

PART 2 WRAP-UP - SPEAK TO LEAD
REFLECT. RESET. REFOCUS.

You've just walked through the sharpest four chapters on OET Speaking you'll find in any book.

You now know:
– The voice isn't just a sound. It's a strategy.
– The criteria don't just score you. They profile your clinical identity.
– Language isn't a filler. It's your frontline.
– Role-plays aren't tests. They're test drives for real patient trust.

Let's cut the fluff:
If you speak like you're unsure, rehearsed, or robotic — you will not walk out with a Band A.
If you lead the conversation — with clinical calm, layered empathy, and structured recovery — you'll leave the examiner no doubt.

THE REALITY CHECK
OET Speaking isn't a performance for applause.
It's a pressure test to see whether your words bring safety, control, and care under fire.
Band B is common.
Band A is commanded.
And now, you've been shown how to command it — profession by profession.

You've trained:
Voice tone as a clinical tool
Phrases that calm, redirect, escalate professionally
Self-scoring against real examiner language
12x role-plays with Band A blueprints

So here's the question:
What happens now?
You reset the game plan. You rehearse with purpose. You lead with language.

REFLECT. RESET. REFOCUS.
Ask yourself these 3 Platinum Prompts — and answer them like someone aiming for Band A:
What's one phrase, tone upgrade, or non-verbal cue I now commit to mastering under pressure?
Which Band A behaviour have I underestimated — and how will I integrate it into every role-play moving forward?
What will I stop doing immediately — because it no longer serves the clinician I'm becoming?

Final Reminder:
This part wasn't about just passing the Speaking sub-test.
It was about learning how to speak like someone who gets remembered — by patients, by colleagues, by examiners.
And you just unlocked that skill.

PART 3 – WRITE TO WIN

Letters That Sound Like They Came from the Ward, Not a Classroom

Let's cut the ceremony.

If your OET Writing still sounds like it was copy-pasted from a grammar textbook — you're not ready.

Because in the real world:
– No referral starts with "Dear Sir/Madam."
– No clinician wants to decode your ramble.
– And no patient has time to wait while you over-explain instead of prioritise.

The examiners?

They're not looking for calligraphy or academic syntax.

They're asking: *Would I trust this clinician's handover under pressure?*
That's the standard. And that's what this part of the book is built for.

The Mission Ahead
Welcome to *Part 3 – WRITE TO WIN*.
You're about to transform your writing from safe and forgettable → to sharp, structured, and worthy of a Band A referral.

Here's what's coming:

Chapter 9. Writing with Professional Authority
You'll drop the student tone and write like a real clinician — with decisions, purpose, and control.
Strategic reframe: Write like it's going on your CV.

Chapter 10. The Writing Criteria Deconstructed
Not just what the scoring guide says — but what it means.
Purpose. Clarity. Conciseness. Tone. Organisation.
Add-on: Band B → A Rubric Snapshots to see exactly what moves the score.

Chapter 11. Case Note Combat Strategy
You'll master the brutal art of triage: What stays, what gets cut, and how it's structured — fast.
Tool drop: The 3-Filter Case Note Cut Test (clinical value / task relevance / reader need).

Chapter 12. Letters by Profession: 12 Tactical Tasks
Not just models — but x12 tactical walkthroughs, with profession-specific insight and coaching commentary.
Extras: Trainer Coaching Margin + Vault access to editable templates.

Why This Matters
Band A writing doesn't sound like a language exam.
It sounds like someone who belongs on the ward.

Band B writing?
Over-explains. Lists without filtering. Gets lost in polite clutter.
This part doesn't just give you writing practice.
It rewires your decision-making.

You'll learn to:
Filter case notes like a diagnostic scan
Structure like a clinical handover
Write for readers — not robots or rubrics
Use tone like a scalpel: precise, professional, powerful

Mindset Check Before We Begin
"Would I feel reassured if this letter was about my patient?"
"Would I trust the person who wrote this to take over care?"
If the answer is no — then you've got work to do.

But don't worry.
Part 3 has your back, your brain, and your Band A strategy.

Ready?

Let's write like someone who's already been hired.

Turn the page. Let the scalpel sharpen.
Chapter 9: Writing with Professional Authority — coming up.

CHAPTER 9 - Writing with Professional Authority

Purpose-Driven, Reader-Aware, Band A Referral Power

CHAPTER MISSION
Train candidates to write referral letters that sound like they were written by a clinician with decisions to make — not a student hoping to pass.

LEARNING OUTCOMES
By the end of this chapter, you will:
Demonstrate reader-aware filtering under time pressure
Deliver task-anchored content using clinical tone and priorities
Justify case note decisions based on referral purpose and audience role
Structure a letter that reads with professional confidence, not polite uncertainty
Refine register, tone, and clarity for Band A impression

TACTICAL WARM-UP (PRESSURE PRIMER)
"You have 4 minutes left, and 17 case notes still untouched. What do you cut first?"
"The reader is a specialist. What language insults their expertise?"
"If the examiner skimmed your letter in 20 seconds, what would they notice?"

STRATEGIC ERROR
The Polite Rambler:
Too many candidates write like they're trying to impress an English teacher instead of briefing a colleague.
They include everything. Use safe phrases. Over-explain symptoms already known to the reader.
Band B writes to tick boxes.
Band A writes to transfer care.

TACTICAL TRUTH
Write like it's going on your CV.
Because it is.
Every letter reveals who you are as a professional communicator.
Clear? Trusted.
Cluttered? Questioned.
Band A writing earns trust without explanation. It sounds like someone with real decisions to make.

COMPONENT & CRITERIA BREAKDOWN
OET Sub-Test: Writing

Criteria Focus:
Purpose
Conciseness & Clarity
Genre & Style
Organisation & Cohesion
Language

Band A sounds like:
A clinician writing to another, with full awareness of roles, relevance, and urgency — and without the "training wheels" of excessive courtesy or explanation.

MINDSET REFRAME: THE CLINICIAN'S UPGRADE

"You're not writing a letter.

You're briefing someone who has 20 seconds to decide what happens next."

STRATEGY SECTION – CHKZ TACTICAL INSTRUCTION
CLINICIAN'S CHOICE
The 3 Command Questions (Before Writing a Word):

Why am I writing? (Referral, update, transfer, etc.)

To whom am I writing? (Role, expertise, expectations)

What do they actually need to know? (What changes their next decision?)

PHRASES THAT WIN POINTS

"Thank you for seeing this Patient regarding..."

"She is being referred for further evaluation of..."

"His condition has been managed with..., but..."

"In light of the unresolved symptoms, I would appreciate..."

"I am writing to request continued management of..."

Avoid:

"This Patient is a 49-year-old male who has been experiencing…" (Textbook trap: no filter, no focus.)

"The Patient states that…" (Reader is not a medical student. Cut the diary tone.)

EXAMINER TRIGGER POINT

Red Flag: List Writing.

Dumping all case notes into a chronological mess shows zero filtering.

If your letter reads like a timeline, not a clinical argument — downgrade incoming.

STRUCTURE MODEL – THE CHKZ SNAP
Opening:

Clear, anchored to task (referral/update/discharge)

Core Paragraphs:

Grouped by clinical theme, not random order

Each paragraph = one idea + justification for inclusion

Final Line:

Polite, professional, purposeful

"Thank you for your ongoing care and support."

PROFESSION EXAMPLES
Medicine

"Given the persistent syncope despite medication, I am referring her to you for cardiological assessment."

Dentistry

"She is being referred for extraction of tooth 27, which remains symptomatic following two unsuccessful RCTs."

Physiotherapy

"Although his mobility has improved, residual hip stiffness remains. I would appreciate your further input for targeted rehab."

REAL-WORLD TRANSFER (CLINIC CROSSOVER)

Clear referral writing supports:
Safer handovers
Legal documentation
Reputation management
Patient confidence
Clinical clarity under time pressure

TRAINER NOTES & DIFFERENTIATION

Coach Up: Have Band B writers summarise their letter in 20 seconds. If they can't, clarity is missing.
Coach Down: Use a paragraph scaffold: Topic → Action → Outcome → Relevance
Watchpoint: "Textbook voice" – safe but sterile.

Mini-Rubric:

Band B: Accurate info, but lacks purpose clarity and role relevance
Band A: Sharp, filtered, reader-aware, and confident in tone

TACTICAL APPLICATION ZONE (BLUE-DIAMOND DRILL)

30-Second Summary Challenge
Explain the purpose of your letter — without looking at it — in 30 seconds or less.

Sentence Surgery
Take this:
"The Patient was admitted on 13th Jan with complaints of dizziness and nausea…"
Make it Band A:
"He presented with persistent dizziness; your assessment is requested to investigate possible vestibular dysfunction."
Case Note Cut Drill
Review 20 notes. Keep only 10. Justify each choice aloud to a peer or coach.

PERFORMANCE WRAP-UP

You are not writing to impress. You are writing to transfer care.
Professional authority in OET Writing = clinical control + audience awareness.

SELF-COACHING QUESTIONS

"Would I trust this handover if I were the receiving clinician?"
"Did I write for clarity, or just completeness?"
"How confident do I sound — even if I'm nervous?"

TRAINER CHALLENGE

Give your candidates 2 versions of the same letter. <u>One Band B. One Band A.</u>
Ask: Which would you want written about your mother?

Next Up:
Chapter 10: The Writing Criteria Deconstructed
It's time to decode what the score means — and how to earn every point.

CHAPTER 10 - The Writing Criteria Deconstructed

What the Scores Actually Mean — and How to Earn Every Point

CHAPTER MISSION

Unpack the OET Writing criteria into real-world behaviours so candidates know exactly what the examiner is rewarding — and how to deliver it under pressure.

LEARNING OUTCOMES

By the end of this chapter, you will:

Distinguish between Band B and Band A performance across all 6 criteria

Apply scoring logic to plan, filter, and write smarter

Justify inclusion, structure, and phrasing based on purpose and reader

Adjust tone and organisation for clinical clarity, not classroom approval

Self-assess using high-band markers

TACTICAL WARM-UP (PRESSURE PRIMER)

"If the letter goes straight to the patient's file, would you still include that phrase?"

"You cut 7 notes but kept 1 vague one. Why?"

"How would the examiner know you've met the purpose — without guessing?"

STRATEGIC ERROR

The Blind Folder Approach:

Too many candidates write like they're being marked by an English teacher.

They focus on spelling and paragraphs — but forget clarity, tone, and purpose.

Or they try to "sound formal" and end up writing like it's 1920.

The result?

Letters that meet the word count — but miss the point.

Band B at best. Band C if rushed.

TACTICAL TRUTH

You're not writing to fill space. You're writing to change action.

Band A letters don't just transfer information.

They target the right data, guide the reader's next step, and earn trust.

Clarity is not about simplicity.

It's about relevance under pressure.

COMPONENT & CRITERIA BREAKDOWN

OET Sub-Test: Writing

6 Official Criteria + What They Really Mean:

1. **Purpose**

Band B: The purpose becomes clear by the end

Band A: The purpose is obvious from the opening line

Use: "I am writing to refer/update/request…" in the first 1–2 sentences

2. **Content**

Band B: Some content is included that's not relevant

Band A: Only clinically-relevant, reader-relevant content is included

Use the "Does this change the reader's decision?" test for each case note

3. Conciseness & Clarity
Band B: Verbose phrasing or case-note copying
Band A: Every sentence filtered for message strength and clinical impact
Cut: "The patient was seen by…" → Use: "He was assessed on…"

4. Genre & Style
Band B: Sentence structure is formal but inconsistent
Band A: Reads like professional, purposeful communication
Avoid textbook English. Aim for clinical brevity and tone.

5. Organisation & Layout
Band B: Order of info loosely follows case notes
Band A: Structured by clinical themes, not time
Paragraphs group key data by topic: "Presenting Symptoms," "Management," "Referral Rationale"

6. Language
Band B: Generally accurate, some awkward phrasing
Band A: Fluid, confident, and controlled throughout
Band A tone = crisp, calm, and controlled. Not fancy. Not robotic.

MINDSET REFRAME: THE BAND A SHIFT
"Band B explains. Band A commands."
Band B says, "The patient has been experiencing…"
Band A says, "She presents with…"
Band B says, "He should consider getting an x-ray."
Band A says, "An X-ray is advised to rule out…"

STRATEGY SECTION – CHKZ TACTICAL INSTRUCTION

CLINICIAN'S CHOICE

When reviewing your draft, apply the Band A Filter Grid:

Test It	Band B Habit	Band A Upgrade
Purpose	Delayed or vague opening	Purpose statement upfront
Content	Over-inclusion of past history	Only includes relevant clinical triggers
Clarity	Long, passive sentences	Short, active voice
Style	Classroom phrases	Clinical register
Structure	Timeline paragraphing	Grouped by action & reader need
Language	Unclear transitions	Anchored with connectives: "In view of…", "To this end…"

PHRASES THAT WIN POINTS
"Given the ongoing symptoms…"
"Her condition has been stable since…"
"I would appreciate your input regarding…"
"He is referred for further evaluation and management of…"

Avoid:

"The patient said that she had been…"

"There was a lot of pain for the patient…"

"This is the reason why I am writing this letter…"

EXAMINER TRIGGER POINT

Case-note regurgitation.

If the letter looks like it was typed line-by-line from the notes, the examiner flags it fast.

REAL-WORLD TRANSFER (CLINIC CROSSOVER)

These criteria map directly to what makes real clinical writing safe, readable, and useful:

PURPOSE = Patient safety

CLARITY = Legal defence

STRUCTURE = Team trust

TONE = Interprofessional respect

TRAINER NOTES & DIFFERENTIATION

Coach Up:

Run a "Red Pen" drill. Highlight every line that could be removed. Band A trims the fluff.

Coach Down:

Give scaffold starters:

"Given the recent events…"

"She has responded well to…"

"Please find enclosed the report on…"

Watchpoints:

Politeness ≠ professionalism

Completeness ≠ clarity

"Formal" ≠ clinical

Band B → Band A Snap Rubric:

Criterion	Band B	Band A
Purpose	Indirect or unclear	Frontline and focused
Content	Overload or drift	Clinically filtered
Clarity	Safe but soft	Concise and assertive
Style	Stiff or student-like	Confident and clinical
Organisation	Copy-paste order	Thematic grouping
Language	Mostly accurate	Controlled and natural

TACTICAL APPLICATION ZONE (BLUE-DIAMOND DRILL)

Criteria Strip Test

Give a completed letter — but no band.

Have candidates identify where each criterion was met (or missed).

Then: Predict the score.

Conciseness Combat

Rewrite this:
"The patient came into the clinic and said that she had been feeling very dizzy and nauseous for the past couple of days."

Make it Band A:
"She presents with a two-day history of dizziness and nausea."

Band A Self-Review Prompt
Ask:
"Would the reader need this sentence?"
"Does this phrase guide the next action?"
"If I cut this, would anything important be lost?"

PERFORMANCE WRAP-UP

You now know how you're being scored — and why Band A letters read differently.
They're not just grammatically sound.
They're professionally powerful.

SELF-COACHING QUESTIONS

"Did I write like someone with clinical responsibility?"
"Would I feel briefed or burdened if I received this letter?"
"What criteria do I hit naturally — and which need sharpening?"

TRAINER CHALLENGE

Take a real student letter. Highlight each sentence in colour-coded criteria categories.

Now: Rewrite only what doesn't serve the reader's decision.
Score again. Discuss what changed — and why.

Next Up:
Chapter 11: Case Note Combat Strategy
You've seen the criteria. Now it's time to cut the noise and keep what counts.

CHAPTER 11 - Case Note Combat Strategy

What to Keep, What to Cut, and How to Structure Like a Pro

CHAPTER MISSION

Train you to filter case notes like a clinician under pressure—prioritising relevance, cutting the fluff, and structuring your letter to serve decision-making, not description.

LEARNING OUTCOMES

By the end of this chapter, you will:

Filter clinical notes for purpose-driven writing

Select data based on receiver need, not habit

Structure letters by clinical function, not case note order

Apply the 3-Filter Cut Test to reduce overload

Build reader-ready paragraphs grouped by themes, not time

TACTICAL WARM-UP (PRESSURE PRIMER)

"Imagine the reader only has 30 seconds. Which data do they need to act?"

"Would you say this out loud on a ward handover?"

"What will the examiner penalise more—missing one mild symptom or including three irrelevant ones?"

STRATEGIC ERROR

Chronological Copying = Clinical Clutter

Candidates panic and start copying every detail from the case notes, in order.

The result?

A letter that's exhaustive, not effective.

A Band B wall of words with no message clarity.

The reader gets lost. The examiner ticks down.

TACTICAL TRUTH

You're not reporting events. You're briefing a colleague.

Band A performers do one thing better than everyone else:

They filter the chaos and shape the meaning.

That's what this chapter trains you to do—quickly, surgically, and with strategic intent.

COMPONENT & CRITERIA BREAKDOWN

OET Sub-Test: Writing

Primary Criteria Addressed:

Content (Is this relevant?)

Conciseness & Clarity (Does this serve a clinical function?)

Organisation & Layout (Can the reader follow this?)

MINDSET REFRAME: THINK LIKE A BRIEFING OFFICER

"In clinical writing, less is more—if the less hits hard."

STRATEGY SECTION – CHKZ TACTICAL INSTRUCTION

THE 3-FILTER CASE NOTE CUT TEST

Run every case note through these three filters:

FILTER 1: Clinical Relevance
Ask: Does this note affect the reader's next action?
Keep:
Primary symptoms
Diagnoses
Red flags or deterioration
Actions needed from the recipient
Cut:
Patient background not relevant to current issue
Lifestyle info that doesn't impact treatment
Family details unless clinically critical

FILTER 2: Reader Relevance
Ask: Would this reader need this info to act?
Example:
You're writing to a physiotherapist.
Keep: mobility issues, pain description, balance tests.
Cut: dietary notes, past unrelated surgeries.

FILTER 3: Purpose Alignment
Ask: Does this support the purpose of referral/update/management?
If yes → rephrase and include.
If not → delete.

CLINICIAN'S CHOICE: STRUCTURE BY THEMES, NOT TIMELINE

Weak Paragraphing (Band B):
1st Paragraph = Admission details
2nd = Symptoms
3rd = Treatment history
4th = Plan

Band A Upgrade: Group by message priority

Paragraph Focus	Typical Content	Why It Works
1. Referral Purpose	"I am writing to refer…"	Sets the mission early
2. Present Condition	Symptoms, urgency, concern	Reader sees what's active
3. Relevant History	Only filtered, necessary background	Context without clutter
4. Treatment Summary	Management to date	Prepares for next steps
5. Call to Action	Requested action, follow-up	Ends with direction

PHRASES THAT WIN POINTS
"Of note, she has had…"
"This was managed with…"
"In view of the persistent symptoms…"
"Your evaluation is appreciated regarding…"

"He is referred for further management of…"

EXAMINER RED FLAG:
Copy-paste syndrome.
If the letter mirrors the note sheet line by line, the examiner clocks it—and drops the score.

REAL-WORLD TRANSFER (CLINIC CROSSOVER)
Effective case-note filtering mirrors real ward communication:
Clear purpose → less time wasted
Thematic structure → faster decision-making
Reader-relevant data → better patient outcomes
This isn't just test strategy.
It's clinical literacy.

TRAINER NOTES & DIFFERENTIATION

Coach Up:
Have advanced learners argue for exclusion. Force a justification for every note they cut.

Coach Down:
Group case notes into columns: Must Include / Maybe / Cut
Discuss each choice and map it to the letter's purpose.

Watchpoints:
"More" is not "better"
Structure = trust
Relevance beats volume every time

Trainer Strip:
Use a coloured marker code when editing learner letters:
Green = Critical info
Yellow = Useful but optional
Red = Cut it — it's fluff

TACTICAL APPLICATION ZONE (BLUE-DIAMOND DRILL)
Live Note Filtering Drill
Give students a raw case note set.
5 minutes: Apply the 3 Filters.
Then:
Circle what stays
Cross what goes
Highlight 1–2 "maybe" entries
Pair up. Justify each.

Rebuild & Restructure
Take a poorly structured sample letter.
Identify the paragraph logic
Regroup the info into new thematic sections
Rewrite only the opening sentence of each paragraph with Band A clarity

PERFORMANCE WRAP-UP

Case notes are not a checklist.

They're a data dump—and your job is to extract the signal from the noise.

A Band A writer is a decision architect:

They plan the reading journey

They lead the clinical eye

They write for the next move, not for the marks

SELF-COACHING QUESTIONS

"Did I write what mattered—or just what was there?"

"Would a colleague thank me for how I structured this?"

"Did my letter act like a scalpel—or a shovel?"

TRAINER CHALLENGE

Bring two letters to the table—one too long, one too vague.

Dissect the difference.

Use the 3 Filters live with your group.

Then: rebuild the paragraph logic together.

Next Up → Chapter 12: Letters by Profession

The strategy is in place. Time to apply it across all 12 OET professions—profession by profession, letter by letter.

Chapter 12 – Letters by Profession: 12 Tactical Tasks

Trainer Coaching Margin and Vault Template Unlocks

Mission Brief: Deliver strategic, profession-specific writing under pressure — with precision, purpose, and clinical tone.

LEARNING OUTCOMES (Scoring Objectives)
By the end of this chapter, learners will be able to:
Deliver high-band, profession-specific letters using targeted clinical language.
Prioritise and structure case notes into reader-relevant letters under time pressure.
Demonstrate tone, clarity, and conciseness across a range of patient, procedure, and practitioner contexts.

TACTICAL WARM-UP (Pressure Primer)
"You have 5 minutes left. You've written too much. What do you cut — and what do you keep?"
"Your letter is being reviewed by the Head of Department — not your trainer. How would you write it differently?"

STRATEGIC ERROR
Trap: Writing "generically" to save time.
Why it fails: It dilutes professional credibility, reduces clarity, and misses reader relevance. Band B lives in the vague. Band A lives in the exact.

TACTICAL TRUTH
Write like it's going in your clinical portfolio.
Band A letters sound like they belong in real files — sharp, specific, and structured. This isn't creative writing. It's clinical correspondence.

COMPONENT & CRITERIA BREAKDOWN
Test Part: Writing Sub-Test
Criteria Mapped: Purpose, Content, Conciseness, Genre/Tone, Organisation, Language
Band A Sounds Like: Reader-first decisions, clinical register, surgical language cuts, accurate sequencing.

Mindset Reframe: The Clinician's Upgrade
"Write like someone's care depends on it — because it might."
This isn't about passing a writing test. It's about proving your communication is safe, credible, and reader-ready under pressure.

CHKZ TACTICAL INSTRUCTION
Each of the following 12 sub-sections provides a complete:
Profession-specific prompt
High-Band model letter
Commentary breakdown (Why this works)

Trainer Coaching Margin (for classroom / 1:1 use)
Vault Unlock Link (access to editable templates)

1. **Nursing**

Scenario: Post-op patient requiring wound care handover
Focus: Prioritisation of complication history + discharge clarity
Trainer Margin Tip: "Don't list everything. List what matters post-op."

2. Medicine
Scenario: Referral to neurologist for seizure workup
Focus: Clinical tone, red-flag symptom escalation
Trainer Margin Tip: "Cut lifestyle fluff — focus on neurological concern and progression."

3. Dentistry
Scenario: Referral to oral surgeon for impacted molars
Focus: Procedure background + urgency indicators
Trainer Margin Tip: "Use dental-specific terms, not general descriptors."

4. Pharmacy
Scenario: Medication review following polypharmacy flags
Focus: Rationalising medication list + highlighting risk
Trainer Margin Tip: "Avoid over-describing each medication. Link drugs to issues."

5. Physiotherapy
Scenario: Ongoing rehab handover post-knee surgery
Focus: Mobility milestones + patient compliance
Trainer Margin Tip: "Sequence therapy stages — don't just describe exercises."

6. Veterinary Science
Scenario: Referral to ophthalmologist for recurring canine conjunctivitis
Focus: Species-appropriate language + behavioural impact
Trainer Margin Tip: "Clinical clarity trumps owner emotions."

7. Dietetics
Scenario: Referral for obesity intervention with comorbidities
Focus: Link diet history with health deterioration
Trainer Margin Tip: "Say what matters — not what they ate on Tuesday."

8. Occupational Therapy
Scenario: Discharge planning post-stroke
Focus: Home safety adaptations + ADL support
Trainer Margin Tip: "Keep OT goals clear — safety, function, independence."

9. Optometry
Scenario: Referral for diabetic retinopathy
Focus: Eye exam summary + visual impact
Trainer Margin Tip: "Be clinical, not descriptive — trust the test terminology."

10. Podiatry
Scenario: Referral for diabetic foot ulcer management
Focus: Progression, healing status, and risks
Trainer Margin Tip: "Clinical + chronological = Band A clarity."

11. Speech Pathology

Scenario: Child with delayed speech — referral to paediatrician
Focus: Developmental timeline + intervention attempts
Trainer Margin Tip: "Make the child the subject — not the carer's stress."

12. Radiography

Scenario: MRI referral for suspected spinal stenosis
Focus: Summarise findings, justify imaging
Trainer Margin Tip: "State the reason. Build the rationale."

REAL-WORLD TRANSFER (CLINIC CROSSOVER)

Every letter is a patient record. If it's vague or verbose, care decisions suffer. Writing with professional authority is a clinical responsibility — not just a test skill.

TRAINER NOTES & DIFFERENTIATION

Coach up by focusing on reader relevance and compression of information
Coach down by modelling Band A vs Band B excerpts
Peer tip: Let learners reverse-engineer from a Band A letter
Rubric Snap: "Does this letter sound like it came from a ward, not a worksheet?"

TACTICAL APPLICATION ZONE (Blue-Diamond Drill)

Case Note Triage (pick top 3 + justify)
Rewrite Weak Paragraphs (Band B → A upgrade)
30-sec Verbal Summary Challenge
Timed Letter Structuring Drill (Bullet Points → Paragraphs in 12 mins)

PERFORMANCE WRAP-UP

You now have strategic templates across 12 professions.
You've seen what a clinically confident letter sounds like.
You know what to keep, cut, and clarify.

Self-Coaching Questions:

"Did I write for the reader — or to impress the examiner?"
"What part of my writing lacks authority — and how will I fix it?"
"Could another clinician act on this letter confidently?"

Trainer Challenge:

Pick a profession outside your own. Deliver a Band A letter with full clinical register.

PART 3 – WRITE TO WIN

Letters That Sound Like They Came from the Ward, Not a Classroom

WRAP-UP: REFLECT, RESET & REFOCUS

You've just completed the written gauntlet.
You now know that OET writing isn't about flowery grammar or textbook perfection — it's about clinical credibility, reader clarity, and decision-driving structure.
From understanding what professional writing really looks like, to dissecting criteria, slicing case notes with precision, and finally delivering Band A performance under pressure — you've seen the difference between fluff and function.
These last four chapters weren't about how to write.
They were about how to communicate like someone who belongs in the system — not just someone trying to pass it.

WHAT THIS PART TAUGHT YOU:
Chapter 9: That authority isn't a tone — it's a by-product of purpose, clarity, and audience awareness.
Chapter 10: That each OET criterion has hidden landmines — and knowing what separates Band B from Band A helps you sidestep them.
Chapter 11: That not all case notes deserve to survive — and tactical triage is a must.
Chapter 12: That writing changes by profession — but the standard doesn't. Excellence is universal. So is strategy.

Clinician's Reframe
"Write it like it's going in the patient's file — not your notebook."
This part wasn't about writing exercises.
It was about your professional evidence trail — how you present clinical facts, how you build trust through tone, and how you communicate with colleagues who don't have time to decode waffle.

CHKZ TACTICAL TRUTH
Your writing should:
Respect the reader's time
Protect the patient's care
Reflect your professional self
When it doesn't — Band B.
When it does — Band A, every time.

Now Reset the Mission
You're not writing to "sound good."
You're writing to be clear, credible, and clinically aligned.

That means:
Cutting the fluff
Owning your tone
Writing like you already work there

3 Reflection Prompts
"If my letter were handed to a busy senior clinician — would they thank me or bin it?"
"Where have I been writing like a student, not a professional — and what will I change today?"
"Which 3 words describe how I want my writing to feel to the reader?" (Choose from: clear, concise, authoritative, respectful, informative, polished, decisive)

Next Mission:
Part 4 – READ FOR CONTROL

Because reading isn't passive — it's how clinical minds scan, filter, and act fast under fire. Time to turn comprehension into command.

Shall we proceed?

Ok, c'mon then – turn the page ☺

PART 4 – LANGUAGE THAT COMMANDS

Strategic Grammar, Tone, and Structure for Respect & Clarity

There's a reason some candidates sound instantly professional — and others sound like they're reading from a student script.

It's not fluency.
<u>It's control</u>.

Control over tense.
Control over tone.
Control over language that does the job, not just fills the air.

This part of the book isn't about passing grammar tests. It's about commanding professional respect with every sentence you write or speak.
Because in OET — and in the real world — grammar isn't for showing off.
It's for clarifying risk, transferring care, and sounding like you know exactly what you're doing.

WHAT YOU'LL MASTER IN THIS PART:

Chapter 13 – Grammar That Pulls Its Weight
The real-world use of grammar under clinical pressure. Tense control. Passive voice. Clarity under time stress.
Includes: Tense Timing Toolkit for each sub-test.

Chapter 14 – Vocabulary That Earns Respect
How to speak with register. The words that land with professionals. The synonyms that sound strategic, not scripted.
Bonus: "Professional-sounding swaps" flash list.

Chapter 15 – Say It Better: Tactical Upgrades
How to level up weak, vague, or casual language — and make it test-proof and clinic-ready.
Includes: Drill & Kill weak-to-strong mapping exercises.

WHY THIS MATTERS
If your grammar is sloppy — you lose clarity.
If your words are informal — you lose credibility.
If your transitions are weak — your structure collapses.
Band A isn't just about what you say.
It's about how you say it under pressure.

THE CLINICIAN'S UPGRADE
"Speak like someone will quote you."
"Write like it's going in a medical handover."
"Choose words that move care forward — not just fill space."
This part of the book builds your linguistic reputation — the way you sound, the way you come across, the way you earn trust with every sentence.

CHKZ STRATEGIC TRUTH

You don't need complex language.
You need clinical control over the language that matters.

Ready?
Let's make sure your grammar carries weight, your vocabulary earns respect, and your phrases upgrade your entire presence — before, during, and after the test.

Turn the page. Let's sharpen your command.

CHAPTER 13 – GRAMMAR THAT PULLS ITS WEIGHT

Tense Control. Passives. Clarity Under Pressure.

Includes: Tense Timing Toolkit per sub-test

CHAPTER AIM
To train candidates to use grammar not as decoration — but as a clinical decision-making tool.

LEARNING OUTCOMES
By the end of this chapter, learners will be able to:
Demonstrate accurate tense control across all sub-tests
Deliver passive constructions to prioritise patient over provider
Structure statements that reduce risk and boost clarity
Filter out redundant grammar that muddies professional tone

TACTICAL WARM-UP
– A nurse says: "The doctor see the patient yesterday."
– You're writing a letter about a procedure that took place last week — what tense must dominate?
– Mid-speaking test, you accidentally say, "I was tell her to rest..." — how do you recover?

STRATEGIC ERROR
Using grammar like decoration, not direction.
Grammar isn't about sounding clever.
It's about guiding understanding under pressure.
The moment grammar becomes vague, tense becomes slippery, or structure becomes bloated — meaning collapses.

TACTICAL TRUTH
Good grammar isn't perfect. It's purposeful.
Band A grammar drives meaning forward — fast, clear, confident.
Not flowery. Not robotic. Just clean and clinical.

COMPONENT & CRITERIA BREAKDOWN
Speaking & Writing Sub-tests
Criteria hit: Linguistic accuracy, grammatical resource, coherence
Band A sounds like: Precision. Flexibility. Recovery when needed.
Under pressure: Clean subject–verb alignment, time-anchored tenses, tone-sensitive structures

MINDSET REFRAME: THE CLINICIAN'S UPGRADE
"Speak like your sentence will be typed into the patient's record."
"Write like your grammar is timestamped."
"Use tenses like a scalpel — not a crayon."

CHKZ STRATEGY – TACTICAL INSTRUCTION

THE 3 QUESTIONS THAT CONTROL YOUR TENSE
Ask before you write or speak:
When did this happen?
Is it still relevant?

Who is affected now?

Band C default: Overuse of present perfect. Jumbled timeline.
Band A upgrade: Anchor to time — use past simple for completed, present perfect for impact, future for planning.
"The procedure was completed on Monday. The patient has since reported mild discomfort."

THE CLINIC LOVES PASSIVES — HERE'S WHY
Passive voice focuses on what happened, not who did it.
Active: "We gave her antibiotics."
Passive: "Antibiotics were administered."
Safer
More professional
Keeps focus on patient, not provider
Use it strategically, especially in Writing and clinical explanations.

CLARITY STRUCTURES: USE THESE
"It is important to note that…"
"The patient was advised to…"
"There is no indication of…"
"The results suggest…"
These stem-style openers build clinical authority and structure your response.

TENSE TIMING TOOLKIT — SUB-TEST SNAPSHOTS

Sub-Test	Tense Focus	Use Example
Speaking	Present Simple / Future	"You will be referred…"
Writing	Past Simple / Passive	"He was diagnosed with…"
Listening Part A	Past Simple	"She complained of…"
Reading Part C	Present Simple (reporting ideas)	"The author states…"

REAL-WORLD TRANSFER (CLINIC CROSSOVER)
Correct tense = legal clarity.
Correct structure = safe shift handover.
Correct voice = professional trust.
A mistimed verb could suggest a missed diagnosis or a falsified record.

TRAINER NOTES & DIFFERENTIATION
Coach Up: Reinforce timeline questions, passive rewrites
Coach Down: Build tense awareness with colour-coded timeline drills
Assessor Watchpoints: Inappropriate use of present perfect; missed passive cues
Peer Coaching Tip: Swap examples and correct each other's tenses aloud

Mini-Rubric Snap:

Band B	Band A
"She is come hospital."	"She came to the hospital yesterday."
"We take blood test."	"A blood test was taken."

TACTICAL APPLICATION ZONE (BLUE-DIAMOND DRILL)

Decision Point Response

Q: **Patient asks,** "What did the doctor say yesterday?"
Band C: "He say… about medicine…"
Band A: "The doctor said that your prescription was adjusted."

Sentence Rewrites
Rewrite: "We give her the painkillers last night."
"Painkillers were administered last night."

Timed Phrase-Mapping
Give learners 60 seconds to convert 3 active to passive clinical phrases under time pressure.

PERFORMANCE WRAP-UP
You're not being marked for grammatical elegance.
You're being marked for grammatical control.
And your patient — or examiner — needs clarity more than cleverness.

REFLECTION CHECKPOINT
"Do my tenses anchor the timeline, or confuse it?"
"Am I using passives where they add clinical clarity?"
"Would my grammar earn me professional respect in a real handover?"

Next up: Vocabulary That Earns Respect.
Because if grammar is the skeleton — vocabulary is the face your message wears.

CHAPTER 14 – VOCABULARY THAT EARNS RESPECT

Register. Collocations. Synonyms That Land.

Includes: "Professional-Sounding Swaps" Flash List

CHAPTER AIM
To train candidates to sound competent, credible, and clinical — every time they open their mouth or pick up a pen.

LEARNING OUTCOMES
By the end of this chapter, candidates will:
Demonstrate use of profession-appropriate collocations and register
Deliver language that reflects clarity, safety, and respect
Filter out casual or vague vocabulary under pressure
Replace common words with clinical equivalents that reflect Band A tone

TACTICAL WARM-UP
– Would you say "The man got worse" in a handover?
– What sounds more professional: "He felt bad" or "He reported ongoing discomfort"?
– Does "She's doing OK" work on a discharge letter?
No. No. And no.

STRATEGIC ERROR
Using general English in a professional domain.
Words like "stuff," "bad," "thing," "OK," and "get" have no place in a Band A performance.
They don't serve clarity. They don't serve precision.
They sound lazy. And worse — they sound unsafe.

TACTICAL TRUTH
Every word earns (or loses) trust.
Band A vocabulary doesn't show off.
It shows up — with clinical precision and professional tone.

COMPONENT & CRITERIA BREAKDOWN
Sub-tests: Speaking, Writing
Criteria hit: Appropriateness of language, lexical resource, tone
Band A sounds like: Calm, precise, professional, adapted to the context
Under pressure: Learners filter for accuracy, not fluency alone

MINDSET REFRAME: THE CLINICIAN'S UPGRADE
"Speak like your message will be acted on."
"Write like someone else will make a decision based on your words."
"Words are tools. Choose the right one."

CHKZ STRATEGY – TACTICAL INSTRUCTION

PHRASES THAT WIN POINTS: THE 'UPGRADE' RULE
For every vague word you know, have a stronger substitute ready.

Let's rewire them.

Casual	Clinical Upgrade
"get better"	"recover / improve"
"thing"	"symptom / condition / factor"
"a bit bad"	"mild discomfort / moderate pain"
"okay"	"stable / within normal limits"
"took"	"was administered / was prescribed"
"feeling funny"	"experiencing dizziness / disorientation"
"bad reaction"	"adverse response / hypersensitivity"

CLINICIAN'S CHOICE:

"Instead of 'He got worse,' say 'His condition deteriorated.'"
"Instead of 'She felt bad,' say 'She reported nausea and fatigue.'"

COLLOCATIONS THAT CLINICALLY FIT

Band C = single-word vocabulary.
Band A = phrase-level control.
You don't just "take medicine."
You administer a dose, prescribe a course, monitor the response, adjust the treatment.

Medical collocation clusters:

Function	Collocations
Symptoms	present with, report, experience, describe
Treatment	initiate, continue, discontinue, respond to
Medication	administer, prescribe, adjust, increase/decrease
Follow-up	scheduled for, referred to, advised to attend

REGISTER MATTERS

OET = Clinical. Not casual. Not academic.
"You need to take the meds or you might get worse."
"It is important that you adhere to the prescribed medication to prevent deterioration."
"I think it's fine."
"There are no current concerns." / "The patient appears stable."

TACTICAL DRILL: FLASH SWAP CHALLENGE

Give learners 60 seconds to upgrade casual into clinical.

You Say	Upgrade
"He felt bad"	"He reported persistent pain"
"She's doing okay"	"She is currently stable"
"He took the meds"	"The medication was taken as prescribed"
"It's a small thing"	"It appears to be a minor concern"
"She got worse"	"Her condition deteriorated"

REAL-WORLD TRANSFER (CLINIC CROSSOVER)

In real clinical handover, your words become someone else's next move.

Wrong word = wrong action = wrong outcome.

Professional vocabulary isn't pretentious. It's protective.

It safeguards patients, builds trust with colleagues, and reflects your professional identity.

TRAINER NOTES & DIFFERENTIATION

Coach Up: Drill professional paraphrasing in high-pressure role-plays

Coach Down: Visual collocation maps + substitution exercises

Peer Coaching Tip: "You say it, I upgrade it" pair drills

Watchpoint: Band C overuses 'get,' 'do,' 'thing,' or unclear pronouns

Mini-Rubric Snap:

Band B	Band A
"He felt bad"	"He reported severe fatigue"
"She did the test"	"She underwent diagnostic testing"
"It got worse"	"Symptoms worsened over 48 hours"

TACTICAL APPLICATION ZONE (BLUE-DIAMOND DRILL)

30-Second Performance

Give a role-play scene. Learner must describe symptoms, give advice, and explain medication — using only upgraded professional vocabulary.

Rewrite Challenge

Sentence: "The man took the medicine and felt a bit better."

Band A version: "The patient adhered to his prescribed medication and reported a slight improvement."

PERFORMANCE WRAP-UP

Vocabulary is visibility.

It shows the examiner — and your future employer — how clearly you think under pressure.

If your words don't match the setting, your message loses power.

Upgrade. Always.

REFLECTION CHECKPOINT

"Are my words vague or vivid?"

"Do I sound like a clinician, or just a candidate?"

"Would my vocabulary earn respect in a hospital handover?"

Next up: Say It Better — where we weaponise weak phrases and upgrade them until they pass the Band A test. Let's go.

CHAPTER 15 – SAY IT BETTER: TACTICAL UPGRADES

Phrase-Level Rewrites That Earn Points — Fast.

Includes: Drill & Kill Format – Weak-to-Strong Mappings

CHAPTER AIM
To upgrade learner output from vague, casual, or clunky into sharp, clinical, and Band A-ready — under pressure.

LEARNING OUTCOMES
By the end of this chapter, candidates will:
Deliver high-precision phrases under test pressure
Replace common errors with powerful upgrades
Apply transitions, reassurances, and summarising strategies in real time
Recognise and avoid phrases that trigger Band B ceilings

TACTICAL WARM-UP
– "I'll tell the doctor."
– "You need to do the test."
– "That's not good."
These are not Band A phrases.
They're either too blunt, too vague, or too flat to build trust.

STRATEGIC ERROR
Relying on functional English instead of professional English.
Band C sounds transactional. Band B sounds polite.
Band A sounds like leadership.

TACTICAL TRUTH
Clarity + Control + Clinical Polish = Band A.
And it's not about big words.
It's about better words — chosen with purpose.

COMPONENT & CRITERIA BREAKDOWN
Sub-tests: Speaking & Writing
Criteria hit: Appropriateness of Language, Relationship Building, Organisation, Tone

What Band A sounds like under pressure:
→ Reassuring but confident
→ Clear but empathetic
→ Direct but not abrupt

MINDSET REFRAME: THE CLINICIAN'S UPGRADE
"Speak like someone will follow your instructions."
"Write like your letter will guide the next steps."
This isn't English class. This is real-world impact simulation.

CHKZ STRATEGY – SAY IT BETTER (DRILL & KILL)

DRILL 1: WEAK → STRONG

Weak Phrase	Band A Upgrade
"That's not good."	"That is a cause for concern."
"You have to do the test."	"It's important we conduct this test to confirm the diagnosis."
"Don't worry."	"It's completely understandable to feel concerned. Let me explain what we'll do."
"You need to come back later."	"I'd like to schedule a follow-up so we can monitor your progress."
"Take this medicine."	"You'll be prescribed this medication to help manage your symptoms."

DRILL 2: CLINICIAN'S CHOICE — WINNING TRANSITIONS
Use these to steer, summarise, or move the interaction forward.
"Before we continue, may I just check..."
"Let's go over what we've discussed so far."
"There are a couple of options we can consider at this point."
"Would it be okay if I explain that step-by-step?"
"If I've understood correctly, you're mainly concerned about…"

DRILL 3: REASSURANCE THAT FEELS REAL
Avoid robotic responses. Own your voice.

Generic	Professional
"That's okay."	"It's completely normal to feel that way."
"Don't worry."	"Let me walk you through what to expect — that usually helps."
"It's fine."	"There's no immediate danger, but we'll monitor closely."
"Just wait here."	"Please take a seat, and I'll update you as soon as I can."

DRILL 4: CLEARER QUESTIONS THAT BUILD CONTROL
Instead of "Anything else?" →
"Is there anything you've noticed recently that we haven't covered yet?"
Instead of "What's wrong?" →
"Can you describe what you've been experiencing in more detail?"

PHRASES THAT WIN POINTS:
• "Based on what you've told me, it sounds like…"
• "To clarify, are you saying that the pain started two days ago?"
• "That's useful to know. Thank you for sharing."
• "I'll make a note of that for the doctor to review."
• "Let me summarise the main points before we continue."

TACTICAL APPLICATION ZONE (BLUE-DIAMOND DRILL)
Decision-Point Responses
Scenario: A patient seems unsure about the medication.
"Just take it. It's good for you."
"Would it help if I explained how the medication works and why it's been prescribed?"

Role-Play Upgrade
Prompt: You've explained a test, and the patient looks worried.
Band C: "Don't worry. It's just a test."

Band A: "I can see this is a bit overwhelming. Let's go through it together, and I'll answer any questions you may have."

REAL-WORLD TRANSFER (CLINIC CROSSOVER)

Whether it's a colleague on the ward or a patient in distress, the way you say something affects how it's received.
A rushed sentence? Misunderstood.
A vague phrase? Misinterpreted.
A clunky explanation? Leads to mistrust.
Band A communication reduces clinical risk. Period.

TRAINER NOTES & DIFFERENTIATION

Coach Up: Turn learner answers into upgraded models. Use peer review: "Who can say it better?"
Coach Down: Start with 1:1 swaps from weak-to-strong. Use sentence stems.
Watchpoints:
– Overuse of modal verbs without clarity ("Maybe we can…" / "You could try…")
– Repetitive starters ("I think… I think… I think…")
Peer Coaching Tip: Use flashcards with weak phrases. Partner must upgrade them live.

PERFORMANCE WRAP-UP

Band A isn't louder. It's smarter.
You don't impress by sounding robotic.
You impress by sounding ready.
Ready to lead.
Ready to explain.
Ready to step up in high-stakes moments with words that work.

REFLECTION CHECKPOINT

"Did I say what I meant — or just what I could remember?"
"Would I feel reassured if I heard this sentence as a patient?"
"How much of my speaking and writing is still too basic — and what am I upgrading from today?"

PART 4 WRAP-UP — REFLECT, RESET & REFOCUS

Language That Doesn't Just Communicate — It Commands.

Strategic Recap: What This Section Delivered
Over the last three chapters, we didn't just talk about grammar, vocabulary, and phrasing — we re-engineered how you use them under clinical pressure.
We dismantled the myth that accuracy alone earns top scores.
We showed you how clarity, conciseness, and clinical tone drive real Band A performance.
And we upgraded your communication toolkit to match the reality of OET — where every word is a decision, and every sentence signals control.

Key Tactical Upgrades Revisited

From Grammar Gaps to Grammatical Precision
→ You now understand tense timing, passive clarity, and form for function.
No overcomplication. No oversimplification. Just the right structure, at the right time, for the right reason.

From Basic Words to High-Impact Vocabulary
→ You've built a register that earns respect.
You can now swap soft language for stronger synonyms — with collocations and formality calibrated to your profession.

From Weak Phrasing to Tactical Execution
→ You've killed the fluff.
You've rehearsed real-time upgrades.
You've learnt to say less — and mean more.

Clinician's Reframe
You are no longer just trying to "speak English well."
You're now calibrating tone, delivering structure, and commanding clarity — like a high-level healthcare professional with purpose.
This is leadership language.
This is safety language.
This is Band A performance — engineered, not improvised.

What You've Built So Far
A voice that reassures, not rambles
Sentences that structure, not scatter
Grammar that serves the message — not gets in its way
Vocabulary that reflects your clinical judgement, not just textbook knowledge
Every chapter was a drill.
Every drill was a weapon.
You now speak and write like you know what's at stake — and how to lead when the room is watching.

Now Ask Yourself — And Answer Honestly:

"Where am I still clinging to safe, overused language that won't get me beyond Band B?"
"If an examiner read my last letter or heard my last role-play — would they trust me as a professional?"
"What three phrases or grammar choices am I upgrading today to sound like someone who belongs in the room?"

What's Next?
You've got the speaking.
You've got the writing.
You've rebuilt your language from the ground up.

Now it's time to face the next battlefield:
Listening and Reading — under fire.
Where focus drops.
Where detail gets missed.
Where panic costs points.

Let's fix that.

Turn the page. Load the tools. It's time for Band A comprehension.
Let's begin PART 5 – UNDER PRESSURE.

PART 5 – PSYCHOLOGY OF PERFORMANCE

Mindset, Muscle, and Mental Control

This Is Where It's Won or Lost
The grammar's sharp.
The phrases are memorised.
Your letters are clean, tight, and targeted.

But none of it matters if, on the day, your mind betrays you.

Welcome to the part of the book where technical skill meets psychological warfare.
Where anxiety can flatten your fluency.
Where a 60-minute Listening test can undo 6 months of prep — simply because your mental systems crashed under pressure.

OET doesn't just test English.
It tests you.
Your focus. Your calm. Your recovery. Your inner voice when things go wrong.

This section is your performance clinic — where we upgrade your mind like you upgraded your writing.

What This Section Delivers

Chapter 16 – The Chimp and the Clinician
Understand the two brains inside you — and who takes over under pressure.
Learn the fast tools to regain control when panic spikes, energy drops, or test-day doubt creeps in.
Add: Trainer Mental Reset Script for test-day use.

Chapter 17 – OET Is a Stage. You're the Professional.
Learn how belief, posture, and delivery shape perception — and scores.
This chapter is not about faking it. It's about stepping into your clinical identity when it matters most.
Add: Vault Challenge – Band A Voice Simulation.

Chapter 18 – Pre-Test Protocols & Mental Routines
We give you the 24h, 60min, and 5min frameworks to calm your nerves, optimise recall, and walk in ready.
You wouldn't go into surgery without a protocol. Don't walk into OET without one either.
Add: Printable checklists, visual wall prep guides.

Chapter 19 – Communicate Like a Clinician for Life
OET is not the end.
It's your audition for real-world leadership — in OSCEs, interviews, patient care, and beyond.
This chapter closes the loop: your voice, your clarity, your calm under pressure — for life, not just one exam.
Reframe: OET is a clinical leadership test. Act like it.

Why This Section Matters More Than Any Vocabulary List
Most people don't fail OET because they can't speak English.
They fail because their psychology collapses at the exact moment they need composure.

This part of the book builds your internal bandwidth.

So when the test comes, you don't just survive it.
You conduct it.
Like a clinician.
Like a leader.
Like someone who's already made it — because they trained like they belonged there all along.

Turn the page.

It's time to stop hoping you'll be calm.
And start training to command your performance.

Welcome to Part 5 – where Band A begins in the mind.

CHAPTER 16 - The Chimp and the Clinician

Emotional regulation + test-day sabotage control

Add: Trainer Mental Reset Script

CHAPTER AIM (MISSION BRIEF)
Train candidates to override emotional sabotage and perform with composure under pressure.

LEARNING OUTCOMES (SCORING OBJECTIVES)
By the end of this chapter, you will:
Demonstrate emotional control strategies under timed conditions
Deliver task performance despite internal interference
Prioritise self-regulation when under cognitive overload
Structure your test-day mindset like a clinical routine
Filter intrusive thoughts and re-anchor to purpose

TACTICAL WARM-UP (PRESSURE PRIMER)
"It's 2 minutes before the Speaking role-play. You blank out. What do you do?"
"You misheard the Listening prompt. Do you panic, guess, or re-centre?"

STRATEGIC ERROR
Band C Sabotage: Emotion overrides execution.
Stress, fear, or perfectionism hijack the task. Candidates spiral when the unexpected happens.

TACTICAL TRUTH
You're not here to feel ready.
You're here to act ready.
Train your nervous system to perform — not just your memory.

COMPONENT & CRITERIA BREAKDOWN
Test Parts Affected: *Speaking, Listening, Writing, Reading*

Criteria Links:
Clinical Communication Effectiveness
Fluency & Coherence
Tone, Organisation, and Task Completion

What Band A Sounds Like Under Pressure:
Calm even when correcting
Patient when clarifying
Strategic when recovering from error
Voice steady, tone consistent, control unshaken

MINDSET REFRAME: THE CLINICIAN'S UPGRADE
"You don't panic when the patient's stats drop — you pivot and lead."
Apply the same clinical detachment to your exam performance.
It's not personal. It's procedural.

STRATEGY SECTION – CHKZ TACTICAL INSTRUCTION

THE CHIMP MODEL: KNOW YOUR ENEMY

From Prof. Steve Peters' Chimp Paradox model:

Brain Mode	Role	Test-Day Behaviour
Human	Rational Clinician	Calm, strategic, verbal
Chimp	Emotional Hijacker	Doubt, freeze, panic

The Chimp is faster, louder, and wrong.

It triggers when:
A task goes sideways
A word disappears mid-sentence
Another candidate "seems better"

CLINICIAN'S CHOICE: OVERRIDE STRATEGIES
When panic hits, do this:
Physiological Reset (30s max)
Inhale 4, hold 4, exhale 6
Drop shoulders. Unclench jaw. Look down then up.

Say (silently): "This is pressure. Not danger."
Cognitive Pivot
Redirect: "What's the next step I can control?"
Micro-goal: "Speak one calm sentence. That's all."

Anchor phrase: "Clinicians solve. I lead this room."
Recovery Line Ready
"Let me rephrase that."
"Just a moment — I'd like to explain that again."
"What I meant to say was…"
These aren't signs of weakness. They're signs of control.

TRAINER MENTAL RESET SCRIPT
Use this before any mock exam or live OET:
"Breathe.
You are not your fear.
This is a simulation of pressure, not a threat to your worth.
You've trained like a clinician.
Now speak, act, and decide like one.
The goal is not perfection. It's presence.
Band A is a state of composure under disruption.
Lead the moment."

REAL-WORLD TRANSFER (CLINIC CROSSOVER)
The same regulation you train here serves you in:
Emergency debriefs

Emotional family discussions
Interdisciplinary disputes
Medical error disclosures
You're not just passing OET.
You're preparing for real-time calm in high-stakes medicine.

TRAINER NOTES & DIFFERENTIATION

Coach up: Anchor strong candidates in voice-body alignment drills.
Coach down: Use breathing + anchor phrases before each speaking turn.
Assessor watchpoint: Penalise robotic fluency. Reward calm correction.
Peer coaching: Have students narrate their inner voice before, during, and after mock tasks.

Mini-Rubric:

Band B	Band A
Rushes or shuts down under stress	Controls tone and adjusts calmly

TACTICAL APPLICATION ZONE (BLUE-DIAMOND DRILL)
30-Second Crisis Challenge
"You just said the wrong dosage during your role-play. Correct it with calm."
Score for:
Poise
Phrase
Tone recovery

5-Minute Chimp Override Drill
Simulate a mock test, but insert one surprise instruction part-way. Learners must reset, breathe, and continue fluently.

Self-Talk Scripts
Write 3 mental phrases for test-day tension. E.g.:
"Lead the sentence."
"Pause is power."
"One task, one breath."

PERFORMANCE WRAP-UP (CHAPTER PLENARY)
You've learned how to identify, intercept, and override emotional sabotage.
You now own tools to anchor your mind — even when the room spins.
You're not here to perform like a student.
You're here to communicate like a calm, composed professional under pressure.

REFLECTION CHECKPOINT
"When pressure hits, do I freeze or reframe?"
"Can I stay clear even when I stumble?"
"Am I training my inner voice as hard as my vocabulary?"

Next: Chapter 17 – OET Is a Stage. You're the Professional.
Time to build your Band A identity — with body language, tone, and presence.

CHAPTER 17 - OET Is a Stage. You're the Professional.

Role belief, body language, vocal control

Vault: "Band A Voice Simulation Challenge"

CHAPTER AIM (MISSION BRIEF)
Train candidates to perform as confident clinical professionals — using body language, vocal authority, and mindset alignment.

LEARNING OUTCOMES (SCORING OBJECTIVES)
By the end of this chapter, you will:
Deliver role-plays and responses with embodied confidence
Control tone, pitch, and pace to reflect clinical credibility
Prioritise presence, posture, and eye contact under pressure
Structure your speaking like someone others trust
Filter hesitation and over-formality into professional presence

TACTICAL WARM-UP (PRESSURE PRIMER)
"If we muted your test and watched your body only — would you look like a clinician or a candidate?"
"If a patient interrupted you — would your voice drop or hold steady?"

STRATEGIC ERROR
Band C Trap: *The voice shakes. The body closes. The role shrinks.*
Test-takers talk like students. They look unsure.
They perform as someone taking a test — not someone leading a clinical moment.

TACTICAL TRUTH
Band A doesn't wait for confidence. It communicates it — from the first breath.
OET is not an academic oral exam.
It's a simulation of clinical reality.
If you don't look the part, you won't score the part.

COMPONENT & CRITERIA BREAKDOWN
Test Part: Speaking
Criteria Mapped:
Clinical Communication Effectiveness
Fluency & Coherence
Appropriateness of Language
Resources of Grammar & Expression

What Band A Sounds Like Under Pressure:
Pauses intentionally, not nervously
Projects voice with authority, not aggression
Uses professional tone — even when interrupted
Keeps body open, still, and engaged

MINDSET REFRAME: THE CLINICIAN'S UPGRADE

"You're not pretending to be a doctor. You are one."

Now speak like it. Sit like it. Decide like it.

Because Band A doesn't belong to the loudest or the smartest — it belongs to the most composed.

STRATEGY SECTION – CHKZ TACTICAL INSTRUCTION
VOICE COMMAND TRAINING

Voice is your most immediate tool. Train for:

Element	Band C	Band A
Pace	Fast and unsteady	Controlled, clear, varied
Tone	Robotic / unsure	Warm, professional, firm
Volume	Inconsistent	Audible but not loud
Clarity	Rushed or mumbled	Pronounced, intentional

PHRASES THAT WIN POINTS:

"I understand this may be worrying. Let me explain."

"It's important we clarify this before discharge."

"What concerns do you have at this point?"

Each phrase must land — not just exist.

BODY LANGUAGE THAT COMMANDS

Stand or sit like someone whose words carry weight.

Spine straight, chin slightly lifted

Shoulders open — not hunched

Gestures purposeful — not fidgety

Eye contact steady, warm, responsive

Facial expression matching tone: calm, clear, sincere

EXAMINER TRIGGER POINT

If you keep touching your face, crossing your arms, or avoiding eye contact — your Band A disappears. Even with perfect language.

VAULT DRILL – "Band A Voice Simulation Challenge"
Listen to two clips. One is Band C. One is Band A.

Spot the difference in:

Vocal control

Empathy tone

Pausing and emphasis

Then record your own version.

Self-assess using this Band A filter:

Does my voice match the message?

Does my tone reassure without sounding fake?

Would I trust me if I heard this in a real clinic?

REAL-WORLD TRANSFER (CLINIC CROSSOVER)
Everything you practise here upgrades your:

Patient trust levels
Ward communication clarity
Interdisciplinary confidence
Interview and OSCE performance
OET isn't about sounding academic. It's about sounding accountable.

TRAINER NOTES & DIFFERENTIATION

Coach up: Run voice variation drills with intentional emotion shifts
Coach down: Anchor role belief with body posture before each turn
Assessor watchpoint: Tone mismatch (e.g., smiling while delivering bad news)
Peer coaching tip: Use "silent observer" feedback on body posture and eye contact

Band B → A Mini-Rubric:

Band B	Band A
Sounds hesitant or overly formal	Sounds like a peer professional
Body passive or tight	Body intentional and calm
Voice unclear in high-pressure moments	Voice holds steady with clinical tone

TACTICAL APPLICATION ZONE (BLUE-DIAMOND DRILL)

Silent Posture Drill

Stand and face your partner.
No talking. No notes.
Just posture, gesture, and eye contact.
Can they read your clinical calm?

Band A Playback Loop

Record yourself reading 3 Band A phrases.
Listen. Critique. Repeat until you believe the voice belongs to a clinician — not a candidate.

Tone Match Role-Plays

Take 3 emotional patient prompts:

"I don't want this treatment."
"No one explained this to me."
"I'm scared."

Your job: *respond with tone, not just words.*
Score for: empathy, control, recovery.

PERFORMANCE WRAP-UP (CHAPTER PLENARY)

This isn't acting. It's alignment.
You are the professional.
The voice, posture, and tone are your uniform.
Band A doesn't arrive when you know more.
It arrives when you own the room — calmly, clearly, and completely.

REFLECTION CHECKPOINT

"Do I look like the role I'm playing — or like I'm hoping for approval?"

"Would I feel reassured hearing myself speak?"

"What one posture, gesture, or vocal habit will I upgrade this week?"

Next up: Chapter 18 – Pre-Test Protocols & Mental Routines

Let's build the 24-hour, 60-minute, and 5-minute game plan to walk in ready, not rattled.

CHAPTER 18 - Pre-Test Protocols & Mental Routines

24h, 60min, 5min Game Plan for Maximum Control

Add: Printable Checklist + Wall Map

CHAPTER AIM (MISSION BRIEF)
Train candidates to manage their mental bandwidth before test day through clinically aligned, psychologically sharp routines that eliminate chaos and maximise readiness.

LEARNING OUTCOMES (SCORING OBJECTIVES)
By the end of this chapter, you will:
Implement a 3-phase test prep strategy (24hr, 60min, 5min)
Reduce panic by replacing "what if" with "I've got this"
Set internal and external conditions for peak performance
Identify and disrupt unhelpful habits before they sabotage your focus
Establish micro-habits that become automatic on exam day

TACTICAL WARM-UP (PRESSURE PRIMER)
– "What did you do the night before your last exam? Was it strategic or survival mode?"
– "You arrive at the test centre. One candidate is pacing. One is smiling calmly. Which one do you want to be — and why?"

STRATEGIC ERROR
Band C Trap: *Leaving performance to chance.*
They cram last-minute. Skip sleep. Scroll for two hours.
They bring tension into the room — and it leaks into every sentence.

TACTICAL TRUTH
Band A doesn't panic. It prepares.
Nerves are normal. But chaos is optional.
You don't control the prompts — you do control the pilot.

COMPONENT & CRITERIA BREAKDOWN
Test Parts: *All 4 Sub-Tests (Speaking, Writing, Reading, Listening)*

Mapped Criteria:
Clinical Communication Effectiveness
Organisation & Structure (Writing)
Engagement & Confidence (Speaking)
Time Management and Focus (Reading, Listening)

MINDSET REFRAME: THE CLINICIAN'S UPGRADE
"The operating room is cold. The lights are bright. The clock is ticking. And yet… the surgeon is calm."
This isn't just a test.
It's a performance under pressure.
Act like you've been there before — because now, you have a plan.

STRATEGY SECTION – CHKZ TACTICAL INSTRUCTION

24-HOUR PROTOCOL: The Calm Before the Calm
DO:
Review 2 model letters + 1 role-play you're proud of
Print your test-day ID, confirmation, and route map
Pack what you need (snack, pen, ID, water, glasses, anything needed medically)
Revisit your Band A Phrase Bank (not all notes — just the gold)
Walk. Stretch. Sleep early. No alcohol. No new drills.

DON'T:
Do a 3-hour mock and panic if you score low
Scroll TikTok or YouTube endlessly
Argue with anyone
Talk to people who drain your calm

60-MINUTE PROTOCOL: The Pre-Performance Bubble
Before you enter the test site:
DO:
Review your Speaking Role Beliefs (See Chapter 17)
Say 5 Band A phrases out loud to rehearse vocal control
Read one short article out loud for fluency flow
Sit quietly. No social chatter. Breathe. Walk slowly.

DON'T:
Over-analyse past mistakes
Compare yourself to others
Mentally rewrite every letter you've ever written
Second-guess what will come up

5-MINUTE PROTOCOL: Right Before They Call Your Name
You're about to walk in. Now act like it.
DO:
Put your phone away.
Stand tall. Breathe in for 4. Hold for 4. Out for 6.

Repeat this internal script:
"I've trained for this. I will speak with clarity. I will write with purpose. I am ready."
If nerves hit — anchor to task, not feeling. Start planning what you will say first.
Smile. Not because you're happy — but because your face tells your brain what to believe.

TOOLKIT ADDITIONS
PRINTABLE CHECKLIST – 'Band A Prep Map'
Includes:
24-hour checklist
60-minute checklist
5-minute pocket mantra card
Test-Day Packing List

WALL MAP: Band A Behaviour Grid
A visual anchor for your prep space:
Left: "Band C Behaviours"
Right: "Band A Corrections"
Designed to train the subconscious daily

REAL-WORLD TRANSFER (CLINIC CROSSOVER)
These aren't just exam tactics.

They are high-performance routines that scale into:
OSCE calmness
Job interview clarity
Clinical composure during real crises
Self-leadership when others are falling apart

TRAINER NOTES & DIFFERENTIATION
Coach up: Role-play the 5-minute protocol under real pressure
Coach down: Help candidates create one "win script" they can repeat aloud daily
Assessor watchpoint: Pre-test tension visible in vocal strain, sentence rush, posture collapse
Peer coaching tip: "Prep Swap" — exchange calming strategies 24hr pre-test

Band B → A Mini-Rubric Snapshot:

Band B	Band A
Stressed, reactive mindset	Structured, calm mental routine
Erratic focus under pressure	Focused execution
Hoping it goes well	Directing the outcome

TACTICAL APPLICATION ZONE (BLUE-DIAMOND DRILL)

PREP REHEARSAL SCRIPT DRILL
Write and record your own "I'm Ready" script.
Recite it daily for 7 days pre-test.
Rewire your narrative.

GROUND & GROW ROUTINE
Sit
3 breaths
Speak: "Today I will lead the conversation."
Visualise one patient saying: "Thank you, I understand now."
(Do this before every mock.)

24HR MOCK SIMULATION
Live the 24h protocol as if test day is tomorrow.
Rate your calmness. Repeat until you're in control.

PERFORMANCE WRAP-UP (CHAPTER PLENARY)
Band A doesn't rely on luck.
It's a result of layering habits until performance becomes default.

Your mind is your command centre.
Set the system.
Run the protocol.
Own the outcome.

REFLECTION CHECKPOINT
"Have I trained my mind as hard as I've trained my grammar?"
"What part of my prep routine needs to change — tonight?"
"Would my future self thank me for how I'm preparing right now?"

Next: Chapter 19 – Communicate Like a Clinician for Life
This is where OET ends — but your leadership begins. Let's reframe this test as the first step in your real-world command.

CHAPTER 19 - Communicate Like a Clinician for Life

This Was Never Just a Test. It Was a Leadership Audition.

Reframe: OET = Leadership Audition

CHAPTER AIM (MISSION BRIEF)
To convert OET communication skills into real-world clinical influence — across OSCEs *(Objective Structured Clinical Examination)*, job interviews, team briefings, patient consults, and leadership moments under pressure.

LEARNING OUTCOMES (SCORING OBJECTIVES)
By the end of this chapter, you will:
Transfer OET strategies into OSCE, ward, and interview contexts
Use Band A communication traits to lead conversations and de-escalate conflict
Demonstrate the voice, tone, and composure of a high-trust clinician
Align language with role, responsibility, and respect
Reframe every future conversation as a reflection of clinical leadership

TACTICAL WARM-UP (PRESSURE PRIMER)
– "You passed the OET. Tomorrow is your OSCE. Do you still speak like someone being assessed — or like someone in control?"
– "A senior consultant interrupts you mid-sentence. Do you freeze — or redirect the conversation with clinical calm?"

STRATEGIC ERROR
Band C Trap: *Leaving OET language in the test room.*
They pass the test... then revert to filler phrases, defensive tones, or uncertain delivery in real clinical scenarios.
Band B is the minimum to survive.
Band A is the baseline for influence.

TACTICAL TRUTH
The real exam is still coming.
Every job interview. Every OSCE. Every emergency.
Each one asks: "Can I trust you to take charge — with your words, tone, and clarity?"

COMPONENT & CRITERIA BREAKDOWN
Mapped From:
OET Speaking: Clinical Communication, Information Gathering, Relationship Building
OET Writing: Purpose, Tone, Organisation

Real-World Mapping To:
OSCE stations and structured communication tasks
Job interviews (panel, peer, or scenario-based)
MDT briefings, patient escalation, counselling conversations
Leadership presence in clinical and academic settings

MINDSET REFRAME: THE CLINICIAN'S UPGRADE
"Every time you speak, you're either building trust — or losing it."
Whether you're handing over to a colleague or facing a distressed family member, your words carry weight.
Speak like someone who will be quoted.

Write like the referral will shape the next intervention.
Communicate like you're already in the job.

STRATEGY SECTION – CHKZ TACTICAL INSTRUCTION

OET → OSCE CONVERSION MAP

OET Speaking Skill	OSCE Transfer
Empathy phrasing	Patient-centred stations
Signposting	Structured scenario steps
Paraphrasing	Explain results / procedures
Clarifying	History taking, consent
Summarising	Case close, shared decisions

Trainer Drill: Take any OET Speaking role-play. Now turn it into an OSCE-style monologue or interactive simulation.

OET → JOB INTERVIEW TRANSFER
Interviewers clock:
Tone: Do you project calm and capability?
Precision: Do your examples land cleanly?
Empathy: Do you connect without over-sharing?
Leadership: Do you take ownership when describing care?

PHRASES THAT WIN POINTS
– "In that scenario, I remained clinically calm while ensuring the patient felt heard."
– "I used clarification strategies from my training to confirm understanding."
– "I prioritised patient dignity throughout the interaction, which helped de-escalate their anxiety."
– "I led the communication clearly, which supported a safe and timely discharge."
Add your own: Create 5 phrases that blend clinical clarity + personal authority.

OET → REAL-WORLD SCENARIOS
Situation 1: The Family Member in Distress
– OET Skill: Empathy + clarification
– Real Transfer: "I can see this is overwhelming. Let me explain again, simply."

Situation 2: The Junior Team Member Looks Lost
– OET Skill: Signposting
– Real Transfer: "Here's what we're going to do next. I'll walk you through it."

Situation 3: Ward Round Summary
– OET Skill: Summary + clinical tone
– Real Transfer: "This is a 76-year-old male admitted for... current plan is..."
KEY PRINCIPLE:
You're not just relaying information.
You're anchoring safety.
Your clarity becomes someone else's calm.

REAL-WORLD TRANSFER (CLINIC CROSSOVER)

What started as OET prep now becomes your core practice.

– OSCEs respect structure
– Interviews reward confidence
– Patients crave clarity
– Leaders value presence under pressure

Your voice = your leadership signature.

TRAINER NOTES & DIFFERENTIATION

Coach up: Mock interview answers using OET-calibrated phrasing

Coach down: OSCE warm-up using Band A strategy recall

Assessor watchpoint: Does the candidate rely on robotic phrases or flex communication based on context?

Peer coaching tip: Try **"Role-Shift"**: Deliver the same message as if you were (a) a student, (b) a junior doctor, (c) a registrar. Which version commands more trust?

Band B → A Mini-Rubric Snapshot:

Band B	Band A
Polite but vague	Clear, confident, calm
Reads the line	Owns the moment
Repeats safe phrases	Flexes with purpose and poise

TACTICAL APPLICATION ZONE (BLUE-DIAMOND DRILL)

"This Is Who I Am" Introduction Challenge
Imagine your next interview or OSCE opening line.

Write and rehearse it using Band A language:
– Clear role
– Confident tone
– Controlled empathy
– Clinically mature phrasing

Scenario Swap Drill
Take one OET prompt. Now adapt your response to:
– A ward handover
– A formal interview question
– A patient escalation call

Mini-Rubric Use
Self-score using Band B → A Rubric for:
– Clarity
– Tone
– Leadership presence

PERFORMANCE WRAP-UP (CHAPTER PLENARY)

You didn't train to pass a test.

You trained to command clarity in high-pressure environments.

Every interaction from here on — interview, handover, team brief — is a leadership moment.

Speak with presence.

Write with intent.

Communicate like the professional they trust when it matters most.

REFLECTION CHECKPOINT

"What part of my OET performance now forms the backbone of my clinical communication?"

"Would I trust me in a crisis — based on how I speak?"

"Which old habits do I need to retire — so I can lead with clarity, not just pass with grammar?"

PART 5 WRAP-UP

REFLECT. RESET. REFOCUS.

Because Pressure Doesn't Break You — It Reveals You.

WHAT YOU JUST MASTERED:

CHAPTER 16 – The Chimp and the Clinician
You met your inner saboteur — and trained it. Emotional control is now part of your clinical toolkit, not your test-day weakness.

CHAPTER 17 – OET Is a Stage. You're the Professional.
You stopped "doing" the test — and started owning the performance. Voice, stance, pace, tone — they're now tools of calm authority.

CHAPTER 18 – Pre-Test Protocols & Mental Routines
You built a personal system. A TACTICAL WARM-UP. A mental shield. No more showing up to the test hoping for the best.

CHAPTER 19 – Communicate Like a Clinician for Life
You broke the fourth wall. OET is no longer just an exam. It's the rehearsal space for every leadership moment you'll ever face.

THE PSYCHOLOGY SHIFT: BAND A THINKING
This part didn't teach you grammar.
It taught you grit.
The kind that speaks calmly in a chaotic ward.
That doesn't crumble when someone questions your competence.
That rewires fear into readiness.
You're no longer just training for the test.
You're training for everything after it.

WHAT TO DO NEXT:
– Finalise your pre-test mental script (build in visualisation + breathing)
– Rehearse your Band A voice with the Vault Simulation Drill
– Practice real-world transfer (OSCE): deliver a short update, a role-play, and a mock interview — all with the same tone, clarity, and leadership

THE BAND A CLINICIAN WALKS IN READY
Not because they memorised a phrasebook.
But because they've trained their nervous system to operate under fire.
And because they understand this truth:
Pressure is not the enemy. It's your invitation to rise.

3-PART REFLECTION PROMPTS
Answer these honestly — then act.

"What part of my test-day routine needs to become non-negotiable — even in real life?"

"When pressure hits, what's my anchor — breath, phrase, gesture, or mindset?"

"What would change if I spoke like someone already in the job — not just chasing it?"

Next stop: PART 6 – TRAINER STRIPS & TOOLS.

Because high performance isn't just taught — it's trained. Let's give coaches what they need to take this even further.

PART 6 – THE QUIET SKILLS

Reading & Listening: Pressure-Proof Precision

Because What You Miss Could Cost You the Mark — or the Patient.

Let's be blunt.
Most candidates underestimate Listening and Reading.

Why? Because they think "quiet" means "easy."

It's not.

Reading and Listening are the silent assassins of your OET result.
They don't shout. They don't give second chances.
They simply test whether you're sharp enough to catch it the first time — while under time, noise, and mental fatigue.
In the clinic, this matters.
If a patient mentions a red-flag symptom and you miss it — it's not a test failure.
It's a clinical one.
This part trains you for both.

WHY THIS PART NOW?
Originally buried in Part 8, these skills have been moved up for a reason:
You can't score Band A without them.
Even with perfect speaking. Even with flawless writing.
If Listening or Reading drags your average, you're out.
So we brought them forward.
Not as filler tasks.
But as core scoring zones — loaded with tactics, timing drills, and clinical logic.

WHAT YOU'LL MASTER

Chapter 20 – Listening Under Pressure
Notetaking under fire. Part A traps. Part C distraction tactics.
You'll train your ears to catch what matters most — when it matters most.

Chapter 21 – Reading with Surgical Focus
Scan fast. Eliminate fast. Infer with clinical logic.
Because the right answer isn't always the obvious one — but it's always in there if you know how to hunt it.

STRATEGIC ADDITIONS
– "Catch It Before It's Gone" Drill Strip — to sharpen attention and inference in Listening
– Timed "Scan & Infer" Challenges — to simulate Band A-level Reading precision
– Signposted entry points for learners who want to train just one skill ("Just Listening" / "Just Reading")

MINDSET UPGRADE: FROM CONSUMER TO CLINICIAN

These are no longer "passive" skills.

They are diagnostic. Active. Strategic.

You're not just reading words or hearing sounds.

You're interpreting patient cues, flagging danger zones, and triaging information in real-time.

Start thinking like a clinician.

Read like you're writing a referral.

Listen like you're catching the symptom that everyone else missed.

Welcome to Part 6 – The Quiet Skills.

Where silence becomes strength — and precision is your power.

First up: Chapter 20 – Listening Under Pressure.

Because once it's said, it's gone. You either caught it — or you didn't.

CHAPTER 20 - Listening Under Pressure

Catch the Clue. Flag the Risk. Filter the Fluff.

CHAPTER AIM (MISSION BRIEF)
Train candidates to decode, extract, and act on spoken clinical detail under time and cognitive pressure.

LEARNING OUTCOMES
By the end of this chapter, you will:
Demonstrate rapid signal-word recognition across Part A, B, and C
Filter clinically relevant information from distractors
Prioritise and sequence information in real-time
Deliver accurate written responses that map to spoken cues
Stay mentally present and strategically calm under listening pressure

TACTICAL WARM-UP (PRESSURE PRIMER)
– The speaker just gave a medication dose and moved on. What was it?
– You heard three symptoms but only one is relevant. Which one do you write down?
– The audio is still playing. Your pen is stuck. Your brain panicked. What now?

STRATEGIC ERROR
Writing everything = remembering nothing.
Candidates panic-write like court stenographers, missing key terms while drowning in detail.
This leads to information overload, illegible scrawl, or totally blank answers by Part C.

TACTICAL TRUTH
Write for clarity. Listen for priority.
The answer is not everything you hear — it's the one thing that matters most to the clinical outcome.

COMPONENT & CRITERIA BREAKDOWN
OET Listening Sub-Test
Part A: Consultation extraction (scored)
Part B: Workplace snippets (multiple choice)
Part C: Abstract or policy-level discussion (multiple choice)

Scoring Focus:
Clinical inference
Recognising implications
Precision under time
Spelling not penalised — clarity is

What Band A Sounds Like Under Pressure:
– Notes are short, clinical, and accurate
– No repetition
– No hesitation
– No wandering off with irrelevant noise

MINDSET REFRAME: THE CLINICIAN'S UPGRADE

You're not "listening to a recording."
You're processing patient data.
In a real ward, you don't get replays. Neither does the OET.

STRATEGY SECTION – CHKZ TACTICAL INSTRUCTION

🎧 PART A: CONSULTATION EXTRACTION

CLINICIAN'S CHOICE
"Don't write it all. Write what a nurse would chart."

PHRASES THAT WIN POINTS
– "Reports severe chest pain since yesterday"
– "Prescribed 5mg once daily — review in two weeks"
– "Worried about side effects and wants reassurance"

EXAMINER TRIGGER POINT
– Wandering answers that show you didn't filter
– Spelling mistakes that change meaning (e.g. dose vs does)

TIPS:
– Pre-scan the case notes: mentally fill gaps ahead of time
– Track speaker switch — patient's words vs professional's
– Mark abbreviations clearly (e.g. SOB = shortness of breath)

PART B: SHORT WORKPLACE EXTRACTS
This is the "blink-and-you'll-miss-it" part.
Each audio = ~30 seconds. 3 options. Only one answer.

LISTEN FOR:
– Tone of voice (e.g. reassurance, urgency, correction)
– Clinical intention (e.g. update, request, instruction)
– Implication (e.g. policy being enforced, patient being prepped)

TRICK
Distractors often sound factually correct but contextually wrong.

TACTICAL TOOL
– Eliminate 1 wrong choice fast
– Confirm your choice before the next clip starts — no rewinds

PART C: POLICY / PROFESSIONAL DISCUSSIONS

THE DANGER?
Language gets abstract. Pace increases. Accent variation is likely.

LISTEN FOR:
– **Shifts** in opinion ("While we used to... now we...")
– **Emphasis** phrases ("It's crucial to understand...")

– **Contrast** cues ("Unlike previous protocols...")
– Professional **dilemmas** ("The challenge with this is...")

PHRASES THAT WIN POINTS
– "She expresses concern over data security"
– "He supports the updated protocol — less risk, more access"
– "Believes the shortage is due to training gaps, not funding"

TACTICAL APPLICATION ZONE (BLUE-DIAMOND DRILL)

🎧 "CATCH IT BEFORE IT'S GONE" AUDIO STRIP
– **Play 3 clinical clips**: <u>one per part (A/B/C)</u>
– Each is played once
– **Learners must write**:
　1. The key info
　2. Who said it
　3. What it means clinically
Debrief as a class: Who caught what, and why?

REAL-WORLD TRANSFER (CLINIC CROSSOVER)
– Active listening isn't just for exams
– It prevents errors, improves trust, and saves time in real care
– Miss one word? You might miss the whole diagnosis

TRAINER NOTES & DIFFERENTIATION
Start Part A with slowed audio for beginners
Emphasise tone and contrast for Part C at higher levels
Peer-train correction by letting students explain why their partner's answer worked or failed

Mini-Rubric:
　Band B = Safe paraphrase but vague
　Band A = Specific, contextual, and inferential

PERFORMANCE WRAP-UP (CHAPTER PLENARY)
You don't need to hear everything.
You need to catch the right thing — and prove you understood it.
Let the others write everything and panic.
You'll write the answer that scores.

REFLECTION CHECKPOINT
"Am I chasing noise, or identifying signal?"
"Would a clinician reading my answer trust it?"
"What phrase or cue did I miss — and how will I train myself not to miss it again?"

Next up: Chapter 21 — Reading with Surgical Focus
Because your eyes must learn to scan like a scalpel.
No wasted motion. No missed detail. No mercy for distractions.

CHAPTER 21 - Reading with Surgical Focus

Cut the Clutter. Spot the Signal. Move with Purpose.

CHAPTER AIM (MISSION BRIEF)
Train candidates to read under clinical pressure — fast, focused, and with strategic accuracy.

LEARNING OUTCOMES
By the end of this chapter, you will:
Demonstrate timed scanning and inference under pressure
Detect logic traps, decoys, and misdirection
Prioritise keywords with surgical accuracy
Filter clinical relevance from filler
Deliver answers that prove comprehension, not guesswork

TACTICAL WARM-UP (PRESSURE PRIMER)
– You've got 90 seconds to answer a question buried in a wall of words. What's your entry point?
– Two answers seem correct. One is a trap. How do you choose?
– You're tired. The topic's dry. But the clock's ticking. What kicks your brain back into gear?

STRATEGIC ERROR
Passive reading leads to passive scoring.
Many candidates read top to bottom, line by line — like they're enjoying a novel. This is not leisure. This is surgery.

TACTICAL TRUTH
You're not here to read. You're here to extract.
Surgical reading means slicing through text, isolating what matters, and moving fast. Every second counts.

COMPONENT & CRITERIA BREAKDOWN
OET Reading Sub-Test
Part A – Expedited reading (4 short texts, 15 mins)
Part B – Paragraph-level workplace extracts
Part C – Opinion/discussion articles (critical reasoning)

Skills Scored:
Scanning (for specifics)
Skimming (for gist)
Inference (for deeper meaning)
Time management (can't pause the clock)

MINDSET REFRAME: THE CLINICIAN'S UPGRADE
You're not a student reading for comprehension.
You're a clinician skimming a policy update between patients.
Or reviewing an allergy note before prescribing.
Move like it matters — because it does.

STRATEGY SECTION – CHKZ TACTICAL INSTRUCTION

PART A – EXPEDITED READING

TASK: 20 questions. 15 minutes. 4 short clinical texts.
Goal: Rapid location and cross-referencing of key information.

CLINICIAN'S CHOICE
"Don't read the text first. Read the question first."

PHRASES THAT WIN POINTS
– "According to Text C…"
– "Which text mentions dosage adjustment?"
– "What is recommended immediately after diagnosis?"

EXAMINER TRIGGER POINT
– Copy-paste answers (not paraphrased = unclear)
– Wrong text choice (poor scanning)

TIPS:
– Use question keywords to find anchor words in texts
– Box titles = thematic filter
– Use abbreviations to save time (e.g. Txt A = "nut allergy referral")

PART B – PARAGRAPH ANALYSIS
TASK: Workplace communications
Focus: Inference, tone, professional intention

WATCH FOR:
– Shift words (however, although, unless)
– Hidden implications (What's being suggested, not said?)
– Register (Is the policy advisory or mandatory?)

TRAPS TO AVOID:
– Choosing the most technical answer (not always right)
– Getting tricked by factual but irrelevant information

TACTICAL TIP:
– Find the tone. It unlocks the author's purpose.

PART C – OPINION & ANALYSIS
TASK: Two long texts with multiple inference questions
Focus: Argument tracking, viewpoint decoding

DANGER ZONE:
– Exhaustion
– False logic cues
– Skimming too fast and missing opinion shifts

KEY STRATEGIES:
– Underline names, dates, policies
– Track stance changes ("Initially… but later…" = shift)
– Don't get lost in big words. Focus on the message.

TACTICAL APPLICATION ZONE (BLUE-DIAMOND DRILL)

TIMED 90-SECOND SCAN & INFER CHALLENGE
How it works:
– Trainer provides a short clinical paragraph
– Learner has 90 seconds to:
   1. Identify 2 key phrases
   2. Answer 1 inference question
   3. Summarise the tone in 1 word

Why it works:
– Mimics test-day brain pressure
– Trains rapid decision-making
– Reinforces focus on what matters

REAL-WORLD TRANSFER (CLINIC CROSSOVER)
– Clinical reading isn't about pleasure — it's about precision
– Whether it's a faxed note, referral letter, or internal memo, the ability to scan, decode, and decide in seconds keeps patients safe
– Learn this skill here. Save time — or lives — out there.

TRAINER NOTES & DIFFERENTIATION
Lower-level learners = start with 2-minute drills
Advanced learners = add "justify your choice" step
Use group scan challenges: fastest accurate answer wins

Band B → Band A?
   B = selected correctly, but couldn't explain why
   A = chose accurately and strategically

PERFORMANCE WRAP-UP (CHAPTER PLENARY)
Reading is not about absorbing.
It's about extracting.
Surgical readers move with sharpness, speed, and control.
Let others drown in paragraphs.
You'll cut to the core.

REFLECTION CHECKPOINT
"Did I scan with purpose, or read out of habit?"
"Would I be able to justify my answer under pressure?"
"What slowed me down — and how will I sharpen that next time?"

Next: Part 6 Wrap-Up – **REFLECT. RESET. REFOCUS.**

Then? The Final Vault.

One last lock to pick.

Let's finish what you started.

PART 6 WRAP-UP

REFLECT. RESET. REFOCUS.

Reading and Listening Are Quiet Skills — But They Win Loud Points.

CLOSING INTEL: THE SKILLS THEY NEVER SEE COMING
They don't shout.
They don't sparkle.
They don't impress on stage like a well-handled role-play.

But Reading and Listening?
They build your base — and your Band.
These are the silent scorers.
The pressure-sensitive skills that measure not what you say, but what you catch.
They reveal whether you notice detail, infer logic, and track meaning at speed.

Clinicians who fail these components don't fail because they're weak.
They fail because they're unaware.
They underestimate the quiet fight.
They overestimate their instinct.
They get tired, go blind to the traps, and hope for the best.

You won't.

Because you've just built something better:
– Tactical scanning that beats the 90-second clock
– Audio precision that filters noise from signal
– Resilience against test fatigue, logical sabotage, and distractors

YOUR NEW REALITY
From here forward, when you open a reading passage or hear a patient consultation:
– You'll spot the trap before it springs.
– You'll track the pattern, not just the words.
– You'll lock the answer, not guess it.

TRAINER TRIGGER: "STRATEGIC QUIET IS NOT WEAK"
Reading and Listening are not passive.
They are active acts of clinical deduction.
Treat them like they matter — because they absolutely do.

FINAL THOUGHT
Test-day success isn't just what you can say.
It's what you catch before it disappears.
That's what makes you not just a candidate — but a clinician.

REFLECTION PROMPTS

What changed most in how I approach Listening or Reading now?
Where was I coasting, and how will I sharpen my method moving forward?
What's my personal strategy when fatigue hits in the middle of a paper — and how will I snap back into focus?

You've completed the Quiet Skills.
What's next?
The Final Vault.
The toolkit. The blueprints. The execution stage.
Let's take everything you've learned… and weaponise it.

Next Stop → THE FINAL VAULT
Templates. Checklists. Tools. Coaching Kits.
Let's finish loud.

PART 7 – PRACTICE & PERFORMANCE TASKS

Real Tasks. Real Pressure. Tactical Feedback.

Welcome to the battlefield.

No more theory. No more warm-up.

This is the arena where your prep gets pressure-tested.
Where your phrases either land… or limp.
Where your timing, tone, and thought process face live fire.
This part is not for the passive.
It's for candidates who are done "reviewing" and ready to compete.
Done wondering if they're ready — and ready to find out.

What You're About to Face:

Chapter 22 – 12 Speaking Role-Plays with Commentary
You'll get 12 real OET-style speaking prompts — one per profession — backed by sharp commentary, Band B-to-A upgrade guidance, and a Trainer Rubric Tracker that reveals the gap before the exam does.
Built for realism, scored for growth.

Chapter 23 – 12 Writing Tasks with Tactical Annotations
It's not just about writing more. It's about writing what matters.
Each letter task is paired with CHKZ-grade commentary, clarity overlays, and the Structure & Clarity Filter.
See exactly what would raise—or wreck—your score.

Chapter 24 – Strategic Question Banks & Phrase Builders
These aren't generic language lists.
They're curated, tagged, and profession-specific solution sets built for high-pressure moments.
Every section trains recall speed, response accuracy, and tone control.

Chapter 25 – Crash Drills and Survival Sets
Got 10 minutes? Use it.
This chapter is a tactical first-aid kit for last-minute revision, confidence resets, and Band B meltdowns.
Includes:
– Rapid scenario generators
– Emergency transitions
– The Band B Rescue Protocol
– 30-second drill strips to rebuild composure fast

The CHKZ Guarantee:
You won't just practise.
You'll perform under pressure — and be shown why it worked or why it didn't.
Every mistake in this section is a gift.
Every success is a snapshot of what's scalable.

WHY THIS SECTION MATTERS

Because many fail the OET after hours of study...

...simply because they never trained like it was real.

This is your edge.

This is the difference between preparation and performance.

You're no longer studying. You're simulating.

You're no longer just learning. You're leading.

Welcome to the final testing ground before test day.

No excuses. No surprises. No fluff.

Let's execute.

Next Up → **Chapter 22**: 12 Speaking Role-Plays with Commentary

Pressure builds. Let's see what your voice does under fire.

CHAPTER 22 - 12 Speaking Role-Plays with Commentary

Profession-Based. Pressure-Tested. Built to Upgrade.

Includes Trainer Rubric Tracker + Band B→A Commentary Flags

CHAPTER AIM (Mission Brief):
Train candidates to execute high-impact speaking role-plays under time pressure — with Band A control, clarity, and clinical leadership.

LEARNING OUTCOMES (Scoring Objectives)
By the end of this chapter, candidates will be able to:
Deliver structured, purpose-driven role-plays across all 12 OET professions
Demonstrate Band A fluency, tone, and interactional effectiveness
Identify Band B errors and apply Band A upgrades in real time
Structure opening, mid-phase, and closing segments with clinical clarity
Adapt language and empathy based on scenario complexity and patient profile

TACTICAL WARM-UP (Pressure Primer)
"The interlocutor just interrupted your explanation. What do you do?"
"The patient becomes emotional mid-sentence. How do you adjust tone instantly?"
"You've only got 40 seconds left, but the issue isn't resolved. Prioritise. Fast."

STRATEGIC ERROR
Band C–B candidates use polite language but lose control.
They explain at the patient. They ask questions without clinical direction. They sound like learners, not leaders.

TACTICAL TRUTH
The OET Speaking sub-test is a leadership simulation.
You are the clinician. The moment belongs to you.
Empathy ≠ weakness.
Politeness ≠ passivity.
You speak with calm command, not permission-seeking hesitancy.

COMPONENT & CRITERIA BREAKDOWN
Sub-test: Speaking
Focus: Clinical communication under time and performance pressure

Criteria:
Intelligibility
Fluency
Appropriateness of language
Resources of grammar and expression
Relationship building
Information gathering/giving

Band A sounds like this:
– Tone modulated with patient's emotional state
– Transitions clean, confident, purposeful

– Clarification requested without loss of momentum
– Clinical concern present throughout — not hidden behind vague language

Mindset Reframe: The Clinician's Upgrade
"Speak like a professional delivering care — not a candidate seeking a score."
"Your job is not to impress. It's to lead the conversation safely, clearly, and with clinical gravitas."

STRATEGY SECTION – CHKZ TACTICAL INSTRUCTION

CLINICIAN'S CHOICE: Opening Lines That Take Control
"Thanks for coming in today. I understand you're concerned about…"
"Before we begin, I want to reassure you that you've done the right thing…"
"Let's start by clarifying a few details — just so I can help you properly."

PHRASES THAT WIN POINTS
"That's completely understandable — may I explain what's happening and what we can do next?"
"If you're comfortable with it, we can explore a few options together."
"It's important that I explain this clearly — shall I begin?"

EXAMINER TRIGGER POINTS
Avoid:
– Over-apologising
– Over-explaining medical detail the patient didn't ask for
– Repeating phrases like "you know" or "I mean"
– Sloppy signposting ("okay… so…")
Use instead:
– Strategic summaries
– Decisive closures ("Before we finish, is there anything unclear?")
– Empathic recalibration phrases when the patient reacts emotionally

REAL-WORLD TRANSFER (CLINIC CROSSOVER)
These scenarios are not acting games.
They mirror real encounters where:
– A patient is scared, misinformed, or hostile
– Your clarity determines compliance
– Your tone influences outcome
– Your calm prevents litigation

TACTICAL APPLICATION ZONE – The 12 Role-Plays
Each profession gets:
One Realistic Prompt
Model Band A Response
Trainer Commentary Strip
Band B Alert Markers + Suggested Upgrades

MEDICINE
Prompt: Explain the risks and next steps after a suspected DVT.
Band A Marker: "Let me clarify the immediate actions we'll take to keep you safe."

Band B Trap: "It could be dangerous. You must go hospital."
Upgrade: "Because of your symptoms, there's a concern about a clot — which we'll investigate urgently."

PSYCHOLOGY
Prompt: Support a patient showing signs of postnatal depression.
Band A Marker: "It's completely valid to feel overwhelmed — can I ask a few questions to better understand how you've been coping?"
Band B Trap: "You should not worry. Many women feel sad."
Upgrade: "This is more common than many realise — and there are ways we can support you."

DENTISTRY
Prompt: Manage a patient worried about an extraction.
Band A Marker: "Pain control is a top priority — let me walk you through what the procedure involves and how we'll minimise discomfort."
Band B Trap: "Don't worry. It's easy and fast."
Upgrade: "Let me explain exactly what to expect — that usually helps reduce the worry."

RADIOGRAPHY
Prompt: Reassure a patient anxious about an MRI scan.
Band A Marker: "It's completely normal to feel uneasy — I'll be right here and talk you through every step."
Band B Trap: "No need to be scared. It's just a scan."
Upgrade: "You'll hear some noises, but the scan itself is painless — I'll explain as we go."

PHYSIOTHERAPY
Prompt: Motivate a patient who's reluctant to continue rehabilitation.
Band A Marker: "Let's talk about what's been hardest — and see how we can adjust the plan together."
Band B Trap: "You must do it. If not, you won't recover."
Upgrade: "Consistency helps healing — but we can pace it so it works for you."

VETERINARY SCIENCE
Prompt: Discuss post-op care for a dog following a leg surgery.
Band A Marker: "Let's go through the signs to watch for and how to keep your pet comfortable during recovery."
Band B Trap: "Give medicine two time and come back later."
Upgrade: "You'll need to give the medication twice a day — and if you notice any limping or swelling, let us know straight away."

DIETETICS
Prompt: Advise a patient newly diagnosed with coeliac disease.
Band A Marker: "Let's walk through some food swaps — and how to make this manageable day-to-day."
Band B Trap: "You cannot eat bread, cake, or anything normal."
Upgrade: "You'll need to avoid gluten — but there are excellent alternatives we can plan into your meals."

SPEECH PATHOLOGY
Prompt: Explain therapy options for a child with delayed speech.
Band A Marker: "Our goal is to build confidence and communication — and I'll show you how to support this at home too."
Band B Trap: "Your child is slow. We need therapy fast."
Upgrade: "Your child's speech is developing at a different pace — therapy can support progress and ease frustration."

OCCUPATIONAL THERAPY
Prompt: Guide a stroke patient on home modifications.
Band A Marker: "Let's look at ways to keep your daily routines safe, manageable, and as independent as possible."
Band B Trap: "You must change your home or you fall."
Upgrade: "A few adjustments at home can reduce the risk of falling and make movement easier for you."

PHARMACY
Prompt: Counsel a patient about interacting medications.
Band A Marker: "Some combinations can reduce effectiveness — let's double-check what you're currently taking."
Band B Trap: "Don't take with other drugs or it's danger."
Upgrade: "This medicine may interact with others — so it's important we review your full medication list."

PODIATRY
Prompt: Advise a diabetic patient with early signs of foot ulcers.
Band A Marker: "Catching this early means we can prevent complications — I'll show you how to monitor and protect your feet."
Band B Trap: "You are careless with shoes. Now is infection."
Upgrade: "There's some early skin damage — but with the right care now, we can avoid infection."

NURSING
Prompt: Calm a patient refusing a wound dressing change.
Band A Marker: "I understand it's uncomfortable — let's go step-by-step so you know exactly what I'm doing."
Band B Trap: "Don't worry. I just do it quickly."
Upgrade: "It may feel a little uncomfortable, but I'll talk you through each step and we can stop if you need a break."

TRAINER NOTES & DIFFERENTIATION
Coaching Up: Train rhythm and tone using playback. Focus on natural pacing and signposting.
Coaching Down: Start with sentence stems. Use echo drills. Role-play simpler emotions before complex ones.
Assessor Watchpoint: Does the candidate control the middle section of the role-play?
Peer Coaching Tip: Use timed pair drills — 2 mins per segment: opening → info gathering → explanation → reassurance → close.

Band B → A Mini-Rubric:

CRITERION	BAND B BEHAVIOUR	BAND A UPGRADE
Tone	Polite but hesitant	Calm, clear, commanding
Fluency	Some hesitation	Smooth, natural delivery
Clinical Focus	Basic	Direct, confident summaries
Interaction	Reactive	Proactive and adaptive

REFLECTION CHECKPOINT
"Am I taking the lead or following the patient's cues blindly?"
"Do I sound like a candidate — or a clinician who's been here before?"
"Would I feel confident trusting someone who speaks the way I just did?"

Next Up → Chapter 23: 12 Writing Tasks with Tactical Annotations
Because how you document clinical care is as important as how you deliver it.

CHAPTER 23 - 12 Writing Tasks with Tactical Annotations

Model + Debrief Per Profession

Includes: "Structure & Clarity Filter" Overlay

CHAPTER AIM (Mission Brief):
Train candidates to produce purpose-driven, clinically accurate letters that hit the reader's brain in one read — not the bin.

LEARNING OUTCOMES (Scoring Objectives)
By the end of this chapter, candidates will be able to:
Produce reader-ready referral, discharge, and update letters across 12 professions
Apply Band A organisation, tone, and information hierarchy
Filter case notes using strategic triage logic
Annotate model letters for structure, sequence, and scoring insight
Transfer writing control to real-world settings (e.g. SOAP notes, discharge summaries)

TACTICAL WARM-UP (Pressure Primer)
"You've got 5 minutes left, and the last paragraph is a mess. What do you cut — and fast?"
"Your reader is a time-poor professional. Can they grasp your letter in under 10 seconds?"
"If the patient read your letter by mistake, would they trust you more or panic?"

STRATEGIC ERROR
Band B letters often prioritise detail over direction.
They explain. They repeat. They translate notes line by line.
Result? A polite mess.

TACTICAL TRUTH
Band A letters filter before they write.
They're shaped by purpose, driven by reader needs, and trimmed with surgical precision.
→ "Clarity is kindness."
→ "Structure is strategy."
→ "Cut the noise. Lead with need."

COMPONENT & CRITERIA BREAKDOWN
Sub-test: Writing
Focus: Clinical documentation

Scoring Criteria:
Purpose
Content
Conciseness & Clarity
Genre & Style
Organisation & Layout
Language
Band A sounds like this:
– Structured: Intro → key findings → relevant history → next steps
– Clinically filtered: only what the reader needs, nothing more

– Tone-neutral and medically objective

– Uses linking and sequence naturally — not from a textbook

Mindset Reframe: The Clinician's Upgrade

"This isn't an essay. It's your professional signature."

"Write like the next clinician's judgment depends on your letter — because it does."

"If your letter were handed to a medic mid-crisis, would it help or waste their time?"

STRATEGY SECTION – CHKZ TACTICAL INSTRUCTION

CLINICIAN'S CHOICE: Structure That Serves

Template Overview:

Intro = Why Am I Writing?

Summary = What's the current issue?

Background = What's medically relevant?

Request = What do I need the reader to do?

Close = Reassurance and sign-off

Don't list all symptoms.

Don't retell the full case.

Don't be vague about the referral action.

"Structure & Clarity Filter" Overlay

Use this before writing:

Filter	Ask Yourself	Keep or Cut?
Reader Lens	Does this info help the receiving clinician act?	Keep
Time Test	Would I say this if I had 30 seconds to explain?	Cut
Clarity Check	Is this sentence doing real work — or just adding words?	Cut or Reword

TACTICAL APPLICATION ZONE – The 12 Letters

Each task includes:

Writing Prompt (by profession)

Band A Model Answer

Annotated Commentary

Band B Pitfall Flags

Structure & Clarity Overlay

Sample Professions and Highlights:
MEDICINE

Task: Discharge letter for patient post-TIA (Transient Ischaemic Attack).

Band A Snapshot: Chronological sequence, concise findings, clear follow-up directives.

Band B Trap: "Patient came with headache. It was TIA. Gave medication and discharged."

Upgrade: "The patient presented with a transient episode of right-sided weakness and slurred speech, later diagnosed as a TIA. He was commenced on clopidogrel and discharged with neurology follow-up scheduled."

Trainer Margin Note: Don't narrate. Distil. Think like a medic, write like a professional.

DENTISTRY

Task: Referral letter for root canal evaluation after failed conservative treatment.
Band A Snapshot: Diagnosis → intervention → current concern → reason for referral.
Band B Trap: "Patient had filling but still has pain. Please do canal."
Upgrade: "Despite restoration of the lower left first molar (36), the patient continues to experience sensitivity and intermittent pain, suggesting possible pulpal involvement. Endodontic evaluation is recommended."
Trainer Margin Note: Avoid phrases like "please do…" — shift from request to informed clinical referral.

VETERINARY SCIENCE
Task: Referral to specialist ophthalmologist for canine corneal ulcer.
Band A Snapshot: Species/breed, clinical signs, treatment history, escalation justification.
Band B Trap: "Dog has eye ulcer. No better. Send for more care."
Upgrade: "The patient, a 3-year-old French Bulldog, presented with a non-healing central corneal ulcer (OD) unresponsive to topical antibiotics over five days. Referral for advanced ophthalmologic management is indicated."
Trainer Margin Note: Precision in breed, anatomical location, and response timeline builds credibility and trust.

NURSING
Task: Transfer letter to GP following wound debridement for a diabetic patient.
Band A Snapshot: Clearly organised paragraphs (procedure, wound status, current management, follow-up).
Band B Trap: "Patient's wound cleaned. Need to continue dressing."
Upgrade: "Following debridement, the wound is currently managed with daily sterile dressings. Ongoing review is recommended."
Trainer Margin Note: Focus on current care AND what the next provider needs to know. Always pass the baton with clarity.

PHYSIOTHERAPY
Task: Discharge letter for post-operative ACL rehabilitation.
Band A Snapshot: Time markers, outcome-oriented summary, specific progression advice.
Band B Trap: "Patient finish 6 sessions. Better now. Can do more."
Upgrade: "Having completed six supervised sessions, the patient has regained 80% of pre-injury strength and is fit to progress to unsupervised exercises."
Trainer Margin Note: Avoid vague positives. Quantify progress and state the next clinical step clearly.

PHARMACY
Task: Referral to physician due to suspected interaction between prescribed statin and new antibiotic.
Band A Snapshot: Structure = Concern → Evidence → Action requested.
Band B Trap: "He is taking two drugs. Maybe problem. Check it please."
Upgrade: "There is a potential interaction between clarithromycin and the patient's ongoing statin regimen. Review of his current prescription is advised."
Trainer Margin Note: Clinical tone must imply confidence — not guesswork. State risk without panic.

RADIOGRAPHY
Task: Report on an X-ray revealing an unreported rib fracture.
Band A Snapshot: Neutral, observational language. Structured: finding → significance → action.
Band B Trap: "Fracture was there but no one see it. Doctor must know."
Upgrade: "A previously undocumented fracture of the 6th rib (left side) was identified. Further assessment may be warranted."
Trainer Margin Note: Radiographers report. They don't diagnose. Precision + professionalism wins.

SPEECH PATHOLOGY

Task: Progress update for a child with speech delay sent to multidisciplinary team.
Band A Snapshot: Audience-aware: avoid jargon, highlight interventions and observed improvements.
Band B Trap: "Child no speak properly still. Need more therapy."
Upgrade: "Since commencing sessions, the child has increased use of two-word phrases and responds consistently to visual prompts."
Trainer Margin Note: Replace vague negative summaries with observable, measured progress — or justified concern.

OCCUPATIONAL THERAPY
Task: Home safety recommendation report for elderly patient post-stroke.
Band A Snapshot: Concise, organised sections — include justification for all changes.
Band B Trap: "Need to move chair and give grab bar. House not safe."
Upgrade: "Installation of a grab rail is advised to reduce fall risk in the bathroom. Bedside chair repositioning will also improve accessibility."
Trainer Margin Note: Always justify. "Why this matters" is what upgrades you from a description to a clinical communicator.

PSYCHOLOGY
Task: Referral note to psychiatric services for escalating depressive symptoms.
Band A Snapshot: Filters emotion through objectivity. Tracks duration, intensity, and functioning.
Band B Trap: "Patient is sad long time. Not better. Needs help."
Upgrade: "The patient has exhibited persistent low mood, anhedonia, and disrupted sleep for the past 5 weeks, with reduced occupational functioning."
Trainer Margin Note: Emotional symptoms must be reported clinically, not narratively. Filter = Facts + Impact.

PODIATRY
Task: Referral to diabetes clinic due to early signs of foot ulceration.
Band A Snapshot: Timeline → site specifics → concern flag → action recommended.
Band B Trap: "Small wound on foot. Diabetes make it worse. Send to clinic."
Upgrade: "A superficial ulcer (0.7cm) has developed on the lateral aspect of the right foot, with mild erythema. Diabetes review is advised to prevent escalation."
Trainer Margin Note: Size. Site. Status. Stage. Report it like the next clinician depends on your words — because they do.

DIETETICS
Task: Progress report for coeliac patient adjusting to gluten-free diet.
Band A Snapshot: Structure = Baseline → Adaptations → Compliance → Next steps.
Band B Trap: "Patient now don't eat gluten. Still some stomach pain."
Upgrade: "The patient has transitioned to a gluten-free diet and reports improved energy, although occasional abdominal discomfort persists. Food diary review scheduled."
Trainer Margin Note: Outcome and observation must be presented clinically — not casually. Stay professional even when discussing food.

TRAINER NOTES & DIFFERENTIATION
Coaching Up: Run blind-case drills. Give summary cards, not full case notes. Force strategic filtering.
Coaching Down: Use colour-coded templates and visual models. Start with fill-the-gap intros and conclusions.
Assessor Watchpoint: Band B candidates often write everything they saw — not what the reader needs.
Peer Coaching Tip: Let learners swap letters and highlight unnecessary sentences in red. Then rewrite the lean version.

Band B → A Mini-Rubric Snapshot

CRITERION	BAND B BEHAVIOUR	BAND A UPGRADE
Purpose	Vague / delayed	Clear in first line
Structure	Chronological	Hierarchical by reader need
Tone	Informal / emotional	Clinical / neutral
Length	Wordy	Trimmed + focused

REFLECTION CHECKPOINT

"Am I writing for clarity — or to prove I read the case notes?"

"Would I respect this letter if I received it as a professional?"

"Have I removed 20% of what I initially wanted to say — and improved it by 200%?"

Next Up → Chapter 24: Strategic Question Banks & Phrase Builders

Because the questions you ask — and the phrases you own — make or break every task under fire.

CHAPTER 24 - Strategic Question Banks & Phrase Builders

Common Problem-Solving Sets

Includes: By-Profession Tagging System

CHAPTER AIM (Mission Brief)
Arm candidates with a high-performance toolkit of clinical questions, responses, and tactical phrases designed to survive any role-play, letter, or verbal confrontation under test pressure.

LEARNING OUTCOMES (Scoring Objectives)
By the end of this chapter, candidates will be able to:
Deploy precise, profession-specific questions and response strategies
Use high-impact phrases to recover, redirect, or reassure under fire
Structure their language to suit tone, context, and clinical purpose
Avoid vague, repetitive, or robotic formulations
Adapt language banks to real-life interviews, OSCEs, and patient conversations

TACTICAL WARM-UP (Pressure Primer)
"The patient isn't listening. What do you say that reclaims the clinical frame — fast?"
"You've just confused the examiner. One phrase. One sentence. How do you fix it?"
"They're challenging your advice. Can your next words recover the room?"

STRATEGIC ERROR
Band B candidates often memorise scripts.
Result? Flat delivery, mismatched tone, and mechanical phrasing that sounds neither real nor reliable.

TACTICAL TRUTH
Band A candidates don't rely on scripts. They command a toolkit.
Their language is modular. Adaptable. Alive.
→ "Clinical confidence isn't memorised — it's built phrase by phrase."

COMPONENT & CRITERIA BREAKDOWN
Sub-tests: Speaking & Writing
Focus: Clarity, clinical control, lexical precision

Scoring Criteria:
Appropriateness of Language
Linguistic Accuracy
Clinical Tone
Coherence and Flow

Mindset Reframe: The Clinician's Upgrade
"You're not a parrot. You're a professional."
"Speak as if the patient's trust depends on the next sentence — because it does."
"Every phrase is a leadership decision."

STRATEGY SECTION – CHKZ TACTICAL INSTRUCTION
PHRASES THAT WIN POINTS

Language banks are grouped by function, not filler. Each section has tactical purpose and is tagged by profession (etc.).

1. Starting Strong

Purpose: Establish clarity and control in the first 30 seconds.

Function	Phrases	Professions
Opening the Conversation	"Good morning, I'll be taking care of you today."	
Confirming Identity	"Could I check your name and date of birth before we begin?"	
Setting the Agenda	"I understand you're here to discuss [issue]. Is that correct?"	
Framing the Role	"My role today is to assess and explain your next steps."	

2. Eliciting Information (without sounding robotic)

Function: Gather clinical details with empathy and control.

Purpose	Strong Phrasing	Professions
Symptoms	"Could you describe when the discomfort began?"	
History	"Have you noticed any patterns or changes recently?"	
Medication	"Are you currently taking anything for this condition?"	
Mental health	"How has this been affecting your daily routine or mood?"	

3. Delivering Difficult News

Function: Maintain calm, control, and dignity.

Phrase	Purpose	Professions
"I'm afraid the test results do show some concerns."	Clarity without panic	
"There are options we can explore together moving forward."	Supportive reframing	
"Let's focus on what we can manage today."	Grounding the conversation	

4. Recommending Treatment

Function: Move from explanation to decision-making.

Phrase	Function	Professions
"Based on what we've discussed, I'd recommend..."	Directive yet respectful	
"The best course of action at this point would be..."	Clinical authority	
"This approach tends to yield the most reliable outcomes."	Professional reassurance	

5. Handling Resistance or Questions

Function: Recover tone, maintain respect, and redirect.

Trigger	Tactical Response	Professions
Patient unsure	"Would it help if I explained the reasons behind this?"	
Emotional concern	"That's a completely understandable reaction."	
Aggressive tone	"Let's take a moment to work through this together."	
Disagreement	"May I clarify what the recommendation is based on?"	

6. Closing with Clinical Command

Function: End clearly, safely, and professionally.

Phrase	Professions
"If you experience any changes, please contact us immediately."	
"You'll be reviewed again in [timeframe]. Until then, follow the instructions we discussed."	
"Is there anything you'd like me to go over again before we finish?"	All

TRAINER NOTES & DIFFERENTIATION

Up-skill Strategy: Turn lists into role-play challenges. Give students a symptom or complaint — they respond only using tools from the bank.

Down-skill Scaffolding: Use two-option phrases ("Would you prefer X or Y?") to help learners develop fluency.

Peer Challenge: "Pick a phrase. Improve it. Make it shorter, clearer, or stronger."

Band B Flag: Candidates sound too polite or vague. Band A sounds intentional, fluent, and reader-aware.

Tactical Drill – Phrase Upgrade Slam

Give weak Band B phrases. Learners rewrite stronger, smarter versions. Example:

Weak	Tactical Upgrade
"You have to do this test."	"This test will give us critical insight before we move forward."
"You need surgery."	"Surgery would offer the most direct and reliable relief."
"I don't know."	"Let me double-check that and get back to you promptly."

REFLECTION CHECKPOINT

"Do I speak to inform — or to lead?"

"Am I using phrases that sound like I care — and know what I'm doing?"

"Could my language hold under pressure — with a distressed patient, an angry examiner, or a time limit?"

Next Up → Chapter 25: Crash Drills and Survival Sets

Because when everything goes wrong — your language, tone, and clarity still have to go right.

CHAPTER 25 - Crash Drills and Survival Sets

Emergency Tools Under Fire

Band B Meltdown Rescue Kit now included

CHAPTER AIM (Mission Brief)
Equip candidates with real-time rescue strategies when panic sets in, time runs out, or clarity collapses. These are your last-stand tools — built for recovery, composure, and scoring control when everything goes wrong.

LEARNING OUTCOMES (Scoring Objectives)
By the end of this chapter, candidates will be able to:
Recover mid-roleplay or task when memory fails or emotions spike
Deploy structured fallback phrases that buy time and rebuild control
Neutralise Band B meltdown triggers (silence, confusion, emotional derailment)
Self-correct without damaging tone, flow, or confidence
Demonstrate leadership under pressure — even during stumbles

TACTICAL WARM-UP (Pressure Primer)
"You've forgotten the word. Now what?"
"The patient just shouted. Your response determines the tone. Speak."
"You're at minute 3 of the writing task and still stuck. What's your move?"

STRATEGIC ERROR
Band B candidates collapse quietly.
They freeze, mumble, apologise, or repeat themselves. It's not the mistake that breaks the score — it's the absence of recovery.

TACTICAL TRUTH
Band A candidates collapse… but land on their feet.
They use tactical transitions, structured resets, and vocal command to steer back into clarity.
→ "A mistake won't break you — unless you act like it did."

COMPONENT & CRITERIA BREAKDOWN
Sub-tests: Speaking, Writing, Listening
Focus: Fluency, Appropriateness, Organisation

Scoring Criteria:
Clinical Control
Tone & Register
Clarity Under Pressure
Repair Strategies

Mindset Reframe: The Clinician's Upgrade
"You're not being tested on perfection. You're being judged on how you respond when things go wrong."
"Silence isn't safety — it's a score-killer."
"Fall like a leader. Rise like a professional."

STRATEGY SECTION – CHKZ TACTICAL INSTRUCTION

THE BAND B MELTDOWN RESCUE KIT™

Situation 1: You Blank Out
Rescue Phrase:
"Give me just a second to put this clearly."
"Let me rephrase that for clarity."
Use time-buying transitions. Say something — just not 'I forgot'.

Situation 2: The Patient Gets Angry or Emotional
Rescue Phrase:
"I understand this is difficult. Let's work through it step-by-step."
"Your reaction makes complete sense — and we'll find the right approach together."
Use tone to ground the conversation. Lead with calm authority.

Situation 3: Examiner Interrupts or Repeats
Rescue Phrase:
"Let me clarify what I meant there."
"Thanks — I'll explain that a bit more clearly."
Don't panic. Reset the line. Re-deliver the point with confidence.

Situation 4: Time Is Running Out
Rescue Phrase:
"Before we finish, let me quickly review the key points..."
"One final thing I want to make sure you leave with is…"
Sprint to summary. Drop your clearest advice line. Exit like a professional.

Situation 5: Mid-Sentence Confusion
Rescue Phrase:
"Sorry — let me put that another way."
"What I meant to say was…"
Self-correct fast. Clarity matters more than fluency in the moment.

PHRASES THAT WIN POINTS UNDER FIRE

Function	Phrases
Regaining control	"Let's focus on the most important point here."
Reframing emotion	"You've got every right to feel that way."
Re-stating advice	"To be clear, I'd recommend..."
Clarifying confusion	"What I'm saying is…"
Closing fast	"I'll leave you with this key advice…"

THE 90-SECOND WRITING PANIC DRILL
Use when writing stalls. Activate the following:
Patient filter: What do they NEED to know?
Action filter: What's being DONE?
Relevance filter: What's IRRELEVANT? Cut it.

Write the first sentence. Use a safe format:

"Thank you for seeing [patient name], who has presented with…"
Then force one action sentence:
"They have been advised to [action]."
You're now moving. Keep typing.

SPEAKING CRASH DRILL – 30-SECOND RESET STRIP
When things go wrong, say:
"Let's step back and go over that clearly…"
"To clarify, the main issue is…"
"What matters most right now is…"
These reset lines signal control. Examiners take note.

TRAINER NOTES & DIFFERENTIATION
Coaching Tip: Simulate failure moments. Force the learner to recover, not restart.
Up-skilling: Use role-reversal — learner plays examiner and tests resilience lines.
Band A signal: Confident tone even during self-correction. No fluster.
Watchpoint: Avoid "Sorry sorry sorry" syndrome — it burns marks, not wins empathy.

TACTICAL APPLICATION ZONE
Performance Drill
Instructor says "Freeze" mid-task. Learner must:
Recover the line
Redirect the flow
Rebuild fluency in 10 seconds

3 Mistake–3 Recovery Drill
Learner must commit 3 forced errors during the task — but recover each with a tactic from this chapter.

PERFORMANCE WRAP-UP
Crash drills are not just emergency tools.
They are indicators of control, self-awareness, and emotional intelligence.
You don't just pass the OET by being perfect.
You pass by staying professional when it matters most.

REFLECTION CHECKPOINT
"Do I have a fallback line for when I freeze?"
"Can I stay calm when the patient, task, or examiner challenges me?"
"Would my tone inspire confidence — even if I made a mistake?"

Next Up → Part 7 Wrap-Up: Reflect, Reset, and Refocus
Where we tie together performance, psychology, and pressure-proof skills — and get you mentally locked in for your final OET push.

PART 7 WRAP-UP

REFLECT. RESET. REFOCUS.

Where your preparation turns into performance.

You've now faced the drills.
You've walked through real prompts.
You've watched Band B get shredded — and Band A rise from the smoke.
This section was not academic.
It was tactical warfare under timed conditions.
Speaking. Writing. Phrases. Pressure. Panic recovery.
All tested — all trainable.
What you've built in Part 7 is not just "test practice."
You've rehearsed command.

Let's recap your toolkit:
12 Profession-Specific Role-Plays
With scoring commentary, rubric triggers, and trainer strips.
12 Real Writing Tasks with Tactical Annotations
Line-by-line clarity upgrades. Purpose, precision, and tone in action.
Strategic Question Banks & Phrase Builders
High-stakes scenarios + reusable professional phrasing across all OET domains.
Crash Drills & Band B Rescue Kits
Because sometimes what saves you… is what you say after you mess up.

What You've Proven (If You've Done the Work):
You now know what Band A sounds like.
You've written like a clinician.
You've spoken like a leader.
You've recovered like a professional.
And you've trained under the one condition that matters most:
Pressure.

Final Tactical Reframe
"If you can perform when it's messy, you're ready when it's clean."
"Real performance doesn't collapse — it adapts."
"You don't need to be perfect. You need to be commanding."

Reflection Prompts (Do. Not. Skip.)
What's my go-to recovery strategy when a role-play goes off track?
→ Do I freeze, fumble, or reframe with control?
What specific writing habits am I now committed to eliminating — for clarity, not just correctness?
→ (E.g., over-explaining, patient history dumping, robotic tone)
Have I trained enough under real time pressure — or just "studied" OET?
→ What will I change in my next 7 days of prep to close the gap?

NEXT STEP → PART 8: CLINICAL COMMUNICATION THAT LIVES ON

Where test preparation gives way to leadership, trust, and lifelong clinical credibility — inside and beyond the exam.

Let's finish this like professionals.

You know what to do now, right?

Ok then – let's turn that page ;-)

PART 8 – THE MISSION BEYOND

Language is Leadership. This Is Just the Beginning.

So, you've done the drills.
You've faced the mocks.
You've rewritten the phrases.
You've survived the silence, the stress, the self-doubt.

But let's be clear:
OET is not your final goal.
It's just a checkpoint.
The real test? Happens every day.
In every ward. Every referral. Every patient who stares at you, hoping you'll make sense of their pain and their paperwork.
That's the real battlefield.
And the language you've trained here — under fire, under time, under pressure — is the very same language that builds trust, delivers care, and earns respect.

What This Final Part Is — And Isn't
This is *not a goodbye.*
This <u>is a recommitment</u>.

In this final section, we strip everything back to one truth:
If you care enough to train this hard… then care enough to lead that well.
Because the Band A voice isn't just for the role-play.
It's for the patient, the pharmacist, the family, the team.
It's for the next job. The OSCE. The emergency call. The leadership meeting.
It's for the moment you realise your voice can be the calm in someone's chaos.

Chapter Preview
26. **Care to Talk. Care to Lead.**
Final Chapter. Final Oath. Final Unlock.
We close with one last clinical reframe — a challenge not just to pass, but to lead.

You'll see how the skills you've built map directly into:
– High-stakes communication
– Clinical leadership
– Trust-building under pressure
– And long-term credibility
You'll also receive your final CHKZ Oath — the mindset badge that separates those who pass… from those who command.

You've Earned This.
You've shown up.
You've sweated the details.
You've rewired your language.
Now finish strong — not for the certificate…

…but for the standard you now represent.

Final Reminder Before You Enter Chapter 26:
"If you speak clearly, lead calmly, and serve clinically —
then the world will feel safer when you open your mouth."

Let's seal the mission.

Let's write the final line.

Let's speak like it matters — because it does.

CHAPTER 26 - Care to Talk. Care to Lead.

Reframe: Speak like someone will quote you.

Final CHKZ Oath + QR Vault Badge Unlock

CHAPTER MISSION
To transform your OET voice from test survival to clinical leadership — and make every word count beyond the exam.

STRATEGIC ERROR
Mistake: Seeing OET as the end. Speaking just to pass.
Why it fails: It produces "exam mode" language — safe, slow, scripted. It breaks down in real-life stress when a patient collapses, a colleague challenges you, or a senior interrupts with a different plan.

TACTICAL TRUTH
Reframe: Speak like someone will quote you.
Not to impress. To influence.
Real leaders don't memorise Band A phrases.
They earn Band A trust — through tone, timing, and truth.

MINDSET REFRAME
"Your communication is not decoration. It's direction."

From now on, every time you open your mouth in English, assume this:
– Someone is listening who's never heard it said that way before.
– Someone is judging the profession based on how you carry it.
– Someone's safety may depend on your ability to speak fast, think clearly, and calm chaos.

THE CHKZ OATH
Sign it mentally. Speak it daily. Wear it professionally.

"I speak clearly — not because I want to pass —
but because someone needs to understand.
I use my words to de-escalate, direct, and deliver.
I will not confuse speed with strength.
I will not mistake silence for weakness.
I speak to be useful. I speak to lead.
Because I care to talk — and I care enough to lead."

[Vault Badge Unlock]: Scan QR for your downloadable CHKZ Oath Card, printable desk poster, and digital share-badge. Wear the mindset.

STRATEGIC UPGRADE
From candidate… to clinician communicator.
Here's the final upgrade.

You've trained the technical:
– Pronunciation

– Grammar
– Conciseness
– Fluency
– Task completion

Now weaponise the invisible:
– Gravitas
– Calm command
– Empathy under pressure
– Ownership of message and moment

That's what gets remembered.
That's what earns trust.
That's what separates the competent from the credible.

PHRASES THAT WIN POINTS — AND PROFESSIONAL RESPECT
Move from functional to unforgettable:

Band B (Safe)	Band A (Commanding)
"Take your medicine daily."	"This prescription isn't optional — it's your next step."
"You need to rest."	"Rest isn't a suggestion. It's part of your recovery plan."
"Let me explain."	"Here's what you need to understand before we go further."
"I'll refer you to the GP."	"I'm escalating this to your GP so we don't lose time."

Don't lecture. Don't waffle.
Lead the message. Then land it.

CLINIC CROSSOVER
In interviews. In OSCEs. In real-time escalation calls.
This chapter isn't about exam points. It's about power.

When you master the voice of clinical command:
– You get taken seriously.
– You build trust fast.
– You become the adult in the room — not just the one with a badge.

TACTICAL APPLICATION ZONE
30-Second Power Phrase Drill
Say each line aloud — with calm tone and clinical intention.
"I won't rush this. I want to make sure we get it right."
"Here's what's happening — and what happens next."
"You've done the right thing by coming in today."
"This isn't about alarm. It's about action."
"Let's keep you safe. That's the priority now."
Record. Playback. Ask: Would I trust this voice in a crisis?

PERFORMANCE WRAP-UP
You've trained the technical.
Now embed the tactical.

This chapter reminded you:

That leadership starts with language

That passing is not the mission — influence is

That how you speak determines how you're seen

REFLECTION CHECKPOINT

Am I still sounding like a test candidate — or a clinical communicator?

Would a new colleague feel safe following my lead based on how I speak?

What phrase, tone, or silence will I now own differently — because it matters?

This was Chapter 26.

This was the line between the OET you trained for — and the future you're about to walk into.

PART 8 WRAP-UP

REFLECT | RESET | REFOCUS

Because language was never just about language.

You've crossed the final threshold.
This wasn't just the end of a book.
This was the start of your voice upgrade — and your professional shift.
Part 8 reminded you that OET isn't the goal.
It's the gateway.

A pass opens a door.
What you do with that door determines everything next.

You've now seen:
How language isn't just about vocabulary — it's about visibility.
How every phrase reveals your mindset, your message, your mission.
And how every test is just a rehearsal for the real pressure — when people are listening because they trust you to lead.
You are not just a candidate.
You're the next voice of clarity in chaos.
The one who talks in a way that makes people stop — and listen.
Now seal that shift. Speak with stakes.
And own your next room like it matters.

What You Built in Part 8
Reframed OET as a leadership audition
Embedded the CHKZ Oath: speak to serve, not just to score
Learned to be quotable under pressure
Trained tone as a tool of clinical presence
Claimed your future communication role — clinician, coach, leader, model

FROM PASSIVE TO POWERFUL
Passing the OET is a line crossed.
But who you become in the process?
That's the real win.
This chapter wasn't about grammar.
It was about gravity.
And the quiet force of a professional who knows their voice holds weight.

FINAL PROMPTS: REFLECT. RESET. REFOCUS.
"Where in my communication do I still sound like I'm hoping to be understood, instead of ensuring I am?"
"When I speak, do I carry the weight of someone others look to in uncertainty?"
"What phrase, tone, or approach will I now retire — and what new one will I use to signal the professional I've become?"

This was the mission beyond the modules.
And it doesn't end here.

Final reminder: Claim your [Vault Badge + CHKZ Oath Certificate] via QR.

Let the world know — you Care to Talk.

And even more?

You care enough to lead.

CONCLUSION

No More Excuses. No More Guesswork.

You didn't just read a book.
You dissected a battlefield.
You decoded what Band A really takes.
You trained like the result actually matters—because it does.

You now understand:
OET isn't just about language. It's about leadership under pressure.
It's not just about passing. It's about becoming someone worth listening to.
In a test where every word could build—or break—confidence, clarity, or care, **your communication is your reputation**.
Band B may be safe.
Band A is strategic. Commanding. Clinically respected.

YOU'VE SEEN HOW TO:
Structure letters like they'll be used in a real ward.
Speak like someone will quote you in handover.
Read, listen, and respond like someone's safety depends on it.
Shift from textbook rehearsals to tactical control.

WHAT NOW?
You move from reader to performer.
From student to clinician-communicator.
From guessing to knowing.
From hoping to owning your score.

You build a ritual.
You return to the drills.
You sharpen your tone.
You train until Band A isn't a surprise—it's a standard.

Final CHKZ Tools Checklist:
Vault codes downloaded
Band B → Band A mapped
Role-plays rehearsed under pressure
Letters rewritten with ruthless clarity
Mental scripts locked in
Trainer Mode margin flags noted
Reflection questions answered—honestly

CLOSING MISSION PROMPT:
You've read the guide. Now be the guide.
Mentor someone.
Share the drills.
Be the clinician who communicates like it counts.

THE FINAL WORD:
Language is not just a tool.
It is your first act of care.
And when you care enough to speak with precision—
You don't just pass a test.
You change a culture.

See you on the wards.
Speak like you mean it. Lead like someone's watching.

You are now exit-ready.

Welcome to the standard.

EPILOGUE

The Test Was Never the Real Test
The room is quiet now.
No patients, no role-plays, no assessors.
Just you.
Looking back, the OET wasn't just measuring your English.
It was measuring your control.
Your clarity under pressure.
Your ability to make someone feel safe—with words.

What You Faced:
You faced an exam designed not to impress, but to filter.
Not to reward fluency—but to expose fragility.
You passed through it—not by sounding perfect,
But by sounding professional.

What You Proved:
That you can organise chaos.
That you can speak with strength, even when unsure.
That your message won't collapse when someone's life—or confidence—is on the line.

This isn't a textbook win.

It's a career-level signal:
You are ready.
You can be trusted.
You've earned a seat in the room that matters.

What Now?
OET is behind you—but the real arenas are still ahead:
– The confused elderly patient who needs your calm.
– The junior who watches how you speak and learns.
– The family who decides to trust the system because they trusted your tone.

This is your language legacy.
It began in test rooms.
It continues in every shift, every ward, every consultation.

So Walk Forward With:
Confidence—not arrogance.
Precision—not perfection.
Purpose—not performance.

Because clinicians don't just treat.
They teach, lead, reassure, and command—
with words.

FINAL WORD:
You cared enough to train.
Now care enough to lead.
Because from this moment on—
Every conversation is the real test.

Say it like it matters. Because it does.

AFTERWORD

From Test to Testament*: What This Book Was Really About*

This book was never just about the OET.

Not really.

Yes, we broke it down—sub-tests, criteria, scoring mechanics, phrase drills, pressure-proof plans.
Yes, we gave you vaults of vocabulary, strategic frameworks, and performance pathways.

But beneath it all, this was always about something bigger:
Language as leadership.
Communication as credibility.
Pressure as proof of who you really are.

You didn't just read a test guide.
You studied yourself—how you respond to chaos, how you steady your voice, how you shape safety with nothing but a sentence.

If You Made It This Far…

You're not just chasing a Band A.
You're chasing mastery.

You've understood what others don't:
The OET doesn't just sort candidates—
It reveals clinicians.
The kind that patients remember.
The kind that teammates lean on.
The kind that steps forward when others hesitate.

You've Been Trained to:
Speak like someone who will be quoted.
Write like someone who takes responsibility.
Listen like it matters.
Read like you're triaging the truth.

And above all—
To perform when the world around you doesn't wait for you to feel ready.

THE REAL AFTER-EFFECT
If this book did its job,
You're walking away with more than strategies.
You're walking away with standards.
For how you show up.
For how you lead.
For how you use your voice—not just to pass, but to protect.

To the readers who cared to talk—
Now care to lead.
We'll hear it in your voice.
We'll feel it in your presence.
We'll know you came prepared.
Because the real test wasn't English.

It was you—

And how far you were willing to go to make every word matter.

Carry it forward.

APPENDICES – THE TOOLKIT VAULT

Because Talent Is Nothing Without Tools

You've built the skills. Now it's time to sharpen the edge.

This section is not a bonus.
It's a weapons vault.

Every code, every page, every tool in this section has been engineered to back you under pressure — not just in study, but in the clinical arena where hesitation costs trust and unclear speech costs care.

This is where the real professionals live — in systems, not guesswork.
In structure, not vibes.
In clarity, not noise.

Here's what's waiting inside:

Code A1 – Profession Phrase Banks
Tactical fluency, not textbook fluff.
Now mapped with Band B → A upgrades
Drill-ready by function, formality, and tone
Organised by the 12 OET professions

Code A2 – Self-Scoring Rubric Checklists
Don't just study. Study like an assessor.
Trainer-grade flags added for coaching use
CEFR indicators embedded for benchmarking
Ideal for 1:1 reflection or peer feedback circles

Code A3 – Clinical Communication Word Banks
Language that signals leadership, risk, clarity, escalation.
Tone control: from reassurance to urgency
Red flag words for high-stakes encounters
Cultural + clinical appropriateness notes included

Code A4 – 60-Day Tactical Study Plan
Because hope is not a strategy.
Pathways mapped by sub-test
Entry-level adaptations for first-time takers
Includes "pressure drill weeks" and reflection resets

Code A5 – Emergency Phrases Toolkit
Last-minute? Meltdown? This is your grab-and-go.
Built-in drill index
"If stuck, say this" language
Organised by breakdown point (e.g., Role-Play Recovery, Letter Opener Freeze)

Code A6 – Quick-Access Drill Index

The shortcut when your brain's on fire and you've got 8 minutes left.
Now with "Survival Sets for Speaking A"
Fast filter by sub-test, skill, and pressure level
Perfect for final-week prep or micro-sessions

Code A7 – CEFR–OET Reference Guide

Decode the levels. Command the scores.
Visual Band B → A upgrade map
Includes functional language + skill indicators
Backwards mapped for targeted remediation

Code A8 – Grammar Kill List & Tense Timing Toolkit

Because grammar should serve clarity — not cause chaos.
Full CHKZ Kill List of weak, vague, or outdated constructions
Profession-specific tense patterns (e.g., referral vs discharge)
Timing map to match tense with task across OET sub-tests

This Vault exists for one reason:

To turn preparation into performance.
To make sure that when you speak, write, read, or respond — it's not luck.
It's clinical control. Under test conditions. With real-world consequences.

Grab what you need.
Use it like you're stepping into surgery.
And never walk into the test without your tools again.

The test isn't just a challenge.
It's a command post.
This Vault?
Your gear to win.

Code A1 — Profession Phrase Banks

Say What Matters. Sound Like You Belong.

Now Expanded with Band B → A Transitions

Why Phrase Banks Matter
Band B uses language that gets the job done.
Band A uses language that inspires trust, shows clinical leadership, and communicates with precision under pressure.
This isn't about sounding robotic or over-polished.
It's about choosing phrases that signal control, care, and clarity — instantly.

These are not filler lines. These are strategic verbal tools designed to:
Build rapport without waffle
Frame risk and reassurance like a professional
Keep the interaction anchored, even when emotions spike
Reduce miscommunication — especially in high-stakes scenarios
Push you from Band B → Band A under real test pressure

How This Bank Is Organised

Each profession has its own zone:
Medicine   Dentistry   Pharmacy   Nursing   Physiotherapy
Audiology   Podiatry   Speech Pathology   Radiography
Dietetics   Occupational Therapy   Veterinary Science

Each profession's section includes:
Band B Default – common phrases used safely, but generically
Band A Upgrade – advanced versions with tone, structure, and intent
Function Tags – what the phrase does (e.g. Reassure | Redirect | Clarify Risk)
Pressure Points – where to deploy them (e.g. Role-play tension | Writing tone reset)

Sample Upgrade Table (Universal Application)

Function	Band B Default	Band A Upgrade
Reassurance	"Don't worry, it's not serious."	"At this stage, there's no indication of anything severe."
Clarifying Risk	"It might be contagious."	"Given its contagious nature, we'll need to take precautions."
Giving Advice	"You should take this medicine."	"This medication is recommended based on your current symptoms."
Managing Emotion	"I understand you're upset."	"It's completely valid to feel that way given the circumstances."
Redirecting	"Let's do this test first."	"The initial step will be to carry out a focused assessment."

PHRASE BANK SNAPSHOT: NURSING

Function	Band B Phrase	Band A Upgrade
Explain a Procedure	"I'll take your blood pressure now."	"I'd like to check your blood pressure to monitor your response."

Function	Band B Phrase	Band A Upgrade
Empathy	"I know this is hard."	"I appreciate this may be difficult — you're not alone in this."
Clarify Instructions	"Take this pill twice a day."	"Please take one tablet every 12 hours to maintain stable levels."

Band A = Precision + Professionalism + Psychological Readiness
Every phrase here has been tested under pressure.
These aren't just "nicer" versions — they are tools for control, tone, and outcome alignment.

BONUS: Vault Phrase Cards
Scan the QR icon at the top of your profession's section to access:
– Audio phrase drills
– Printable drill cards (Band B → A swaps)
– Flash practice games for trainers and study partners

FINAL WORD
The test doesn't care if your words are "fine."
It rewards clear, confident, and clinically credible communication.
So choose phrases that sound like they came from a practitioner —
Not a textbook.

Proceed to Code A2 → Self-Scoring Rubric Checklists
Because if you can score yourself like an assessor, you can speak like a Band A.

Code A2 — Self-Scoring Rubric Checklists

Score Yourself Like an Assessor. Train Yourself Like a Clinician.

Now includes Trainer Flags + CEFR Alignment Indicators

Why This Matters
Guessing your score is a trap.
Training without a clear scoring mirror leads to stagnation.
This isn't about false confidence or endless second-guessing.
This is about becoming your own examiner, coach, and calibrator.

These checklists are built to help you:
Analyse real performance against Band A–C descriptors
Spot tactical strengths and scoring threats fast
Upgrade isolated elements without losing sight of the full task
Cross-map your current level with CEFR indicators for clarity
Train independently, or with a peer or trainer guiding the session

What's Included in This Code

Each checklist is provided in 2 formats:

Version	Use For
Learner-Friendly Format	Daily drilling, reflection, peer swaps
Trainer Flag Format	Targeted coaching, Band B→A intervention, group sessions

Each format covers:
Speaking
– Clinical control
– Fluency under fire
– Tone, empathy, structure
– Listener engagement + role-play control

Writing
– Purpose, clarity, conciseness
– Reader orientation
– Organisation and logical flow
– Linguistic precision and tone

CEFR–OET Alignment Snapshot

Band A (OET)	CEFR C1+	Commands complex tasks fluently, adapts tone/register to context, leads interaction, structures with purpose
Band B (OET)	CEFR B2	Handles routine communication with occasional lapses, uses standard phrases, may lack precision or impact
Band C+ / C	CEFR B1–	Basic control, effortful expression, limited range, tone often inconsistent with professional scenarios

Use this map to self-locate, then self-level up.

Speaking Sub-Test: Learner Self-Scoring Example

Criterion	What You Did	Yes		No
Tone & Empathy	Used respectful and validating phrases			
Organisation of Information	Grouped advice logically and signposted			
Relationship Building	Built trust with calm, collaborative tone			
Grammar & Vocabulary Range	Mostly accurate, with limited flexibility			
Role-play Management	Redirected patient assertively when off-topic			

Add a reflection note: What will you try differently next time?

Writing Sub-Test: Trainer Flag Format Example

Trainer Flag	Observed	Impact	Next Step
Over-explaining	Yes	Reader fatigue, unclear focus	Apply "Cut Test" from Chapter 11
Passive overuse	Moderate	Reduces urgency + clarity	Use active phrasing for key actions
Strong signposting	Yes	Easy flow, logical structure	Reinforce this habit in future tasks

Use this format in training groups, peer workshops, or mock OET debriefs.

Bonus Vault Link:
– Printable trainer templates
– Editable digital checklists for speaking/writing
– Colour-coded CEFR mapping sheets
– Self-assessment & peer-assessment hybrid versions
Scan QR from Vault badge or download via your Trainer Toolkit companion pack.

FINAL WORD
If you can't measure your level, you can't manage your improvement.
This isn't just self-scoring.
This is self-leadership — in test prep and beyond.

Proceed to Code A3 → Clinical Communication Word Banks
Because the words you choose under pressure aren't just linguistic —
They're clinical tools.

Code A3 — Clinical Communication Word Banks

Say What Matters. Say It Like a Clinician.

Now includes: Tone Escalation + Risk Language Banks

Why This Exists
Language in healthcare is never neutral.
Every word either builds trust, clarifies risk, or creates confusion.
In high-stakes settings, how you say it is as vital as what you say.

This bank isn't a list of random phrases.

It's a clinical toolkit for high-performance communicators who:
Want to sound like they belong in the room
Need to adjust tone for urgency, reassurance, or escalation
Must deliver safety messaging without losing empathy
Are preparing for interviews, OSCEs, or real-life ward leadership

Word Bank Categories
Each section comes in 3 columns:
Band C–B Phrases (Safe but basic)
Band A Upgrades (Strategic, professional tone)
Clinician Commentary (When + why to use)

1. Reassurance Without Overpromising

Basic	Upgrade	Why It Wins
"It's okay."	"At this stage, there's nothing alarming."	Keeps hope grounded in clinical honesty.
"Don't worry."	"I understand your concern — let's focus on what we can manage today."	Validates + redirects with control.
"You're fine."	"Your current observations are stable."	Sounds like a clinician, not a comforter.

2. Escalating Risk — Without Inducing Panic

Basic	Upgrade	Why It Wins
"This is serious."	"This presents a significant clinical concern."	Flags risk clearly without dramatics.
"You need help."	"We'll need to involve another team to support this next step."	Implies structured escalation, not failure.
"You should go to hospital."	"I strongly recommend immediate hospital assessment."	Adds weight, maintains autonomy.

3. Expressing Uncertainty — With Professional Confidence

Basic	Upgrade	Why It Wins
"I'm not sure."	"Let me check that to ensure I give you an accurate answer."	Shifts doubt into accountability.

Basic	Upgrade	Why It Wins
"Maybe."	"At this point, that remains a possibility — we'll monitor closely."	Keeps authority while acknowledging limits.

4. Giving Instructions — Without Sounding Like Orders

Basic	Upgrade	Why It Wins
"You must take this."	"It's important that you take this as prescribed to avoid complications."	Clinical logic, not coercion.
"Don't do that."	"Try to avoid X, as it may interfere with your recovery."	Empowers with rationale, not command.
"Come back tomorrow."	"We'll need to review this again tomorrow to assess progress."	Reinforces follow-up as part of care, not demand.

5. Empathy and Validation Phrases

Basic	Upgrade	Why It Wins
"I know it's hard."	"What you're feeling is completely valid, and we'll take it one step at a time."	Names the emotion and leads forward.
"It's normal."	"Many patients experience similar concerns — you're not alone in this."	Offers clinical solidarity.
"Sorry about that."	"I understand that may have been uncomfortable — thank you for letting me know."	Keeps tone professional, not apologetic.

How to Use This Bank

Highlight your current go-to phrases
Mark the Band A upgrades you're not yet using
Build your own "Top 20 Tactical Phrases" list from across categories

Practise in pairs or solo using the PHRASES THAT WIN POINTS format:
Scenario
Band C attempt
Band A upgrade
Why it wins

Bonus Feature: Tone Escalation Ladder
A printable strip from "Reassuring" → "Neutral" → "Firm Clinical Directive"
Use it to rehearse language shifts under stress or time pressure.

Vault Add-Ons

Flashcard decks: "Band B → A Phrase Drill"
Simulated Role-Play Prompts by Tone Type
Printable peer feedback strip for phrase swaps
Voice Drill Companion: "Say it like a senior. Sound like it counts."

FINAL WORD

Language isn't just how we communicate.
It's how we lead, protect, and heal — or confuse, undermine, and delay.

Train the words now, so you don't scramble for them later.

Proceed to Code A4 → 60-Day Tactical Study Plan

Because elite performance isn't random.

It's mapped.

Code A4 — 60-Day Tactical Study Plan

Train Like You're Going to War — Not Just to Pass.

Includes Sub-Test Pathways + Entry-Level Adaptation Tracks

Why This Exists
Most study plans are either:
Too vague ("Do Speaking on Mondays")
Too crammed ("Cram 4 letters this weekend")
Or not aligned to how clinicians actually learn under pressure.
This plan is different.

It's engineered for strategic performance:
Clinically relevant
Time-calibrated
Profession-sensitive
Sub-test-specific
Whether you're 60 days out or just getting serious now, this plan gives you OPTIONS — not overload.

How It Works
Choose your sub-test priority and your starting tier.

Then follow the 60-Day Route Map tailored to:
Your profession
Your performance pressure zone (e.g. Speaking A panic? Writing letters? Listening collapse?)
Your Band A ambition (Not just "pass")

Entry-Level Track Selector

Band Now	Use This Plan	Why
Strong B	Band A Booster Route	You've got base skills. Now it's about tactical upgrades and timing drills.
Mid B	Core Strategy Route	You need consolidation + 1:1 improvement on structure, tone, and sub-test tactics.
Band C+	Precision Builder Route	Focus on clarity, repair skills, and building up the 4 sub-test cores with structure.

60-Day Masterplan Breakdown
Every week = 5 core focus days + 2 recap/stretch days.
Each day = 60–90 minutes of tactical, high-intensity input

WEEKLY THEMES (ALL ROUTES)

Week	Focus	Tactical Outcome
1–2	Mission Reset + Skills Mapping	Know your Band B traps. Start collecting Band A phrases.
3–4	Sub-Test Deconstruction	Deep-dive into Speaking + Writing scoring criteria and task demands.
5–6	Tactical Rebuild	Implement Band A tools under pressure. Review model answers.

Week	Focus	Tactical Outcome
7–8	Simulation + Strategy Lock	Timed tasks. Mental rehearsal. Performance mindset. Train like it's test day.

Custom Pathways by Sub-Test Focus
Choose based on YOUR weakness.

SPEAKING SURGE PLAN

3 Role-Play Tasks per week (across 3 different professions)
2 Reflection logs with Band B → A comparison
1 Voice Drill with "Command the Conversation" phrasing
1 Peer or trainer feedback task
CEFR Speaking Self-Scoring Tracker (linked in Vault)

WRITING UPGRADE ROUTE

3 Letter Tasks (1 with case note cut test, 1 with Band A overlay, 1 from your profession)
2 Trainer Strip checklists
1 Sentence rewriting session (tactical tone upgrades)
1 Band A model study

LISTENING LASER PLAN

4 audio strips: focus on Part A signal words + B/C inference links
2 "Catch it Before It's Gone" drills
1 peer teaching moment: "Explain what the speaker meant"
1 mistake-mapping session (where do you lose marks?)

READING STRIKE PLAN

3 timed passages (use 90-second Scan & Infer Drill)
2 Logic Trap Review tasks
1 Vocabulary Cluster Builder
1 self-challenge: "Can I explain the distractor and why it's wrong?"

Add-On Study Tools (Vault Links)
Printable 60-Day Wall Calendar
QR access to "Survival Sets for Speaking A"
Daily OET Phrase Builder Flashcards
Crash Drill Simulation Pack (Weeks 7–8)
CEFR–OET Progress Grid

FINAL WORD

You don't rise to the level of your hopes.
You fall to the level of your training.
You've got 60 days. Make them surgical. Make them count.
Proceed to Code A5 → Emergency Phrases Toolkit

Because when pressure hits, autopilot takes over —
…and your autopilot needs Band A language.

Code A5 — Emergency Phrases Toolkit

Say the Right Thing, Right Now — Under Fire.

Now Includes Drill Index for Rapid Deployment

WHY THIS TOOLKIT EXISTS
When the clock's ticking…
When the Patient is confused…
When the examiner's pen pauses mid-note…
Your words must work.
This isn't about elegance.
This is about verbal survival under pressure.
Band A candidates recover fast.
They redirect, de-escalate, clarify — without pausing, panicking, or sounding robotic.
These phrases aren't "nice-to-have."
They're mandatory under fire.

HOW TO USE THIS TOOLKIT
Quick Access Before Role-Plays: Highlight your weak zones (e.g. clarification, reassurance).
In-Task Recovery: Memorise 1–2 default responses per function for fallback use.
Drill in Pairs or Solo: Use the Drill Index below to rehearse by function or profession.
This toolkit is your verbal defibrillator.

STRUCTURE
Each section includes:
Tactical Phrase Bank
Band B → A Upgrade Examples
Memory Hook or Drill Format

EMERGENCY PHRASE ZONES

1. CLARIFYING CONFUSION (Patient / Role-Player)
"Let me just make sure I've understood that correctly..."
"Could you say that another way, just so I'm clear?"
Band B: "What do you mean?"
Band A: "Could you clarify what you mean by that, just to ensure I don't miss anything important?"

2. PAUSING TO THINK / BUYING TIME
"That's a great question. Let me think for a second…"
"Before I answer, let me just double-check something   "
Band B: "Umm… wait… okay…"
Band A: "Let me take a moment to organise my thoughts."

3. REASSURING WITHOUT PROMISING
"I understand your concern, and I'll do everything I can to support you."
"You're not alone in this — let's go through it step by step."
Band B: "Don't worry, it's fine."
Band A: "It's understandable to feel that way, and you've done the right thing by bringing it up."

4. DE-ESCALATING ANGRY OR FRUSTRATED PATIENTS

"I can see this has been incredibly frustrating — thank you for explaining it so clearly."

"Let's work together to sort this out."

Band B: "Calm down."

Band A: "I can see this has affected you deeply. Let's go through it together calmly so nothing's missed."

5. CORRECTING MISINFORMATION (Gently)

"I can understand why you might think that, but actually…"

"That's a common belief, but the evidence shows…"

Band B: "That's wrong."

Band A: "Let me offer some updated guidance based on current clinical standards."

6. ASKING SENSITIVE QUESTIONS

"Would it be alright if I asked something a little personal, just to get a clearer picture?"

"This might be a bit uncomfortable, but it's important for your care — is that okay?"

Band B: "Do you have sex?"

Band A: "Can I ask about your sexual health, just to ensure a thorough assessment?"

7. CLOSING WITH PROFESSIONAL POLISH

"I'll document this and make sure the team is updated."

"If anything changes, please don't hesitate to contact us."

Band B: "Okay, bye."

Band A: "Thanks for your time today — and please let us know if anything's unclear later."

RAPID-USE DRILL INDEX

Function	Drill Prompt	CHKZ Format
Clarify	"Patient gives a vague history."	3-response ladder: confirm, rephrase, check
Reassure	"Patient is anxious about outcome."	Reassure → Reframe → Redirect
De-escalate	"Patient raises voice over delay."	Validate → Decompress → Refocus
Buy Time	"Forgot the term you need."	Delay line + partial redirect
Close	"You're out of time."	Summarise → Invite question → Close professionally

FINAL WORD:

These phrases aren't decoration — they're armour.

When the nerves hit and fluency drops,

when Band B chaos sneaks in —

these words hold the line.

Drill them. Default to them. Deliver with them.

Proceed to Code A6 → Quick-Access Drill Index

Because memorising is one thing — executing under fire is another.

Code A6 — Quick-Access Drill Index

When Pressure's High, the Right Drill Saves the Score.

New Category Added: Survival Sets for Speaking A

WHY THIS INDEX EXISTS
Anyone can study.
Not everyone survives Speaking Part A.
When your brain blanks…
When your voice trembles…
When the timer runs faster than your thoughts…

What saves you?
Muscle memory. Tactical default lines. Drills done cold.
This index isn't for theory.
It's for reaction-level preparation — so you don't think, you respond.

HOW TO USE THIS INDEX
Rotate 2–3 drills per day leading to test week.
Simulate under time: no more than 45–90 seconds per drill.
Speak them out loud — typing doesn't build fluency.

DRILL TYPES IN THIS INDEX

Drill Type	Purpose	Target Area
Survival Sets for Speaking A	Default phrases to rescue test under pressure	Fluency, recovery, reassurance
Band B → Band A Rewrites	Upgrade weak phrases to professional tact	Language control, tone
3-Line Dialogue Drills	Quick verbal exchanges with clarity control	Interaction, clarity, tone
Role-Switch Reframes	Take the patient's concern and respond tactically	Empathy, structure
Timed Recovery Lines	Respond to 5-second panic prompts	Fluency under fire

SURVIVAL SETS FOR SPEAKING A (NEW CATEGORY)
Your emergency go-to responses. Memorise. Deploy. Repeat.

Scenario	Band A Default Line
Patient confused	"Let me explain that another way to make sure it's clear."
You blank on a word	"The term has slipped my mind — but what I mean is…"
Patient emotional	"I can see this is difficult for you — take your time."
You need time to think	"That's an important point. Give me one second…"
Need to correct yourself	"Sorry, I misspoke — what I meant was…"
Closing in a rush	"Before we finish, is there anything still unclear?"

DRILL SET EXAMPLES BY FUNCTION
Band B → A Rewrite Drill
Weak: "You must take the pill."
Strong: "It's important that you take this as prescribed — it's essential for your recovery."

3-Line Dialogue Drill
Trainer: "I don't understand what you said."
You: "Let me rephrase that to make it clearer. What I meant was…"
Trainer: "Okay. That helps."

Role-Switch Reframe Drill
Patient: "I'm scared of what's going to happen."
You: "That's completely understandable — let me walk you through each step so you know exactly what to expect."

Timed Recovery Line Drill
Prompt: "You forget the name of a medication."
Response (in 5 seconds): "I'll need to double-check the name, but it's the medication used to reduce inflammation in this case."

TRAINER TIP
Use this index:
Before class as a warm-up
At the end of class as a performance challenge
In pairs: one gives the crisis, one responds on the spot

FINAL WORD
This isn't about remembering everything.
It's about remembering the right thing — fast.
In the chaos of the test, drills are discipline.
They're your verbal CPR.

Proceed to Code A7 → CEFR–OET Reference Guide
Because knowing what the test wants — and what the real world needs — is where leadership starts.

Code A7 — CEFR–OET Reference Guide

Align. Upgrade. Perform.

Now includes Band B → A Upgrade Map

WHY THIS MATTERS
Most OET candidates aim to pass.
You're not most candidates.
Band B gets you through the door.
Band A gets you remembered, promoted, and trusted.

This guide connects two vital performance lenses:
CEFR (Common European Framework of Reference) – the global language standard
OET (Occupational English Test) – the clinical communication battlefield
Together, they shape how you prepare — and how you show up.

CEFR vs OET — What's the Difference?

Feature	CEFR	OET
Scope	General English (A1–C2)	Clinical English (B to A)
Focus	Language proficiency	Clinical communication
Scoring	Global academic benchmark	Profession-specific pressure score
Benchmark	C1 = Advanced	B = Safe, A = Superior

CEFR–OET Alignment Snapshot

CEFR	OET Band	What It Means
B2	Band B	Safe. Clear. Sometimes robotic.
C1	Band A	Confident. Precise. Clinically agile.
C2	Band A+	Leadership level. Sounds native. Commands the room.

BAND B → A UPGRADE MAP

What to fix, what to finesse, and what to let go.

Category	Band B Sounds Like…	Band A Sounds Like…	Tactical Fix
Tone	Flat or overly formal	Professional + human	Rehearse tone shifts by scenario
Structure	Long, unclear answers	Ordered, strategic phrasing	Use "Signpost + Support + So What" model
Vocabulary	Safe but vague	Domain-specific, intentional	Swap general terms for clinical collocations
Recovery	Avoids repair	Owns and redirects with calm	Drill polite clarification & correction lines
Empathy	Excessive or generic	Balanced, targeted reassurance	Practise emotional calibration by case type
Grammar	Accurate but slow	Accurate + fluent under time	Tense Timing Toolkit + sentence automation

BAND A BEHAVIOURS (CEFR C1/C2 STYLE)

Skill	CEFR Performance Benchmark
Listening	Understands nuance, implied meaning, speaker attitude
Speaking	Adapts tone, controls flow, holds command of room
Reading	Synthesises meaning under time pressure
Writing	Concise, reader-oriented, logically sequenced

EXAMINER TRIGGER POINTS

What Band A sounds like under pressure:
"Let me rephrase that to ensure clarity."
"I appreciate that this may feel overwhelming."
"Let's walk through the next steps together, one by one."

What triggers Band B:
"You understand?"
"I think maybe you should do this."
"It's okay, don't worry." ← (Over-reassurance with no plan)

TRAINER STRIP – HOW TO COACH THE UPGRADE

From B to A:
Target tone + structure before vocab
Simulate fatigue + pressure conditions
Use Band A audio models + real-time rewrites
Anchor feedback to real-world safety and clarity, not just test outcome

FINAL WORD

Passing is a requirement.
Commanding respect is a decision.
CEFR shows you what English can do.
OET shows you what English must do — when it counts.

Proceed to Code A8 → Grammar Kill List & Tense Timing Toolkit
Because when every word matters, grammar must carry weight — not waste time.

Code A8 — Grammar Kill List & Tense Timing Toolkit

Strip the Sloppy. Train for Clinical Precision.

Now includes profession-specific examples for maximum relevance

WHY THIS MATTERS
You don't need to be a grammar nerd.
You need to be grammatically surgical.
Every sentence in OET — spoken or written — is on the clock and under judgment.
Clunky tense choice? Band B.
Passive chaos? Band B.
Unnecessary conditionals, modal overload, or vague time references? Welcome to Band B.
Grammar doesn't win you the score.
But it sure as hell can lose it.

This toolkit gives you two things:
The Kill List – grammar choices that sabotage clinical clarity
The Timing Toolkit – tense rules that help you sound like you're already working on the ward

THE GRAMMAR KILL LIST
Spot it. Stop it. Strip it.

What to Kill	Why It Fails	What to Do Instead
Overuse of conditionals ("If you will…")	Unnatural, ambiguous	Be direct: "You'll need to…"
Random passive overload ("The medicine was being taken…")	Awkward, distant	Use active where clarity matters: "You took…"
Unanchored modals ("You could maybe possibly…")	Doubtful, weak	Use clear clinical verbs: "You'll be advised to…"
Tense inconsistency ("She had went…" / "You are have…")	Grammar breakdown = trust breakdown	Use high-frequency patterns + tense drills
Excessive progressive forms ("She is being vomiting…")	Sounds non-native	Fix form: "She has been vomiting since…"

THE TENSE TIMING TOOLKIT
Say what happened. Say what happens next. Say it like a clinician.

Tense	When to Use	Examples
Present Simple	Routine, current facts	"He takes medication daily."
Present Perfect	Unfinished past with now impact	"She has had a fever since Sunday."
Past Simple	Completed past events	"He fell last night."
Future Simple	Clear future action	"You'll be referred to a specialist."
Present Continuous	In-progress now	"She is recovering well."
Modal + Base Form	Polite advice / clinical suggestion	"You should increase your fluid intake."

PROFESSION-SPECIFIC EXAMPLES
MEDICINE

"The medication was being given yesterday."
"He received the medication yesterday."
"You should maybe take this test."
"I'd recommend you take this blood test to confirm the diagnosis."

PSYCHOLOGY

"You was thinking this too much."
"You've been feeling overwhelmed, which is completely understandable."
"If you talk to someone, you could maybe feel better."
"Speaking with a counsellor might help you process this more effectively."

DENTISTRY

"You are having the pain since Tuesday?"
"Have you been experiencing pain since Tuesday?"
"We maybe will extract the tooth."
"If the infection doesn't improve, we may need to extract the tooth."

OPHTHALMOLOGY

"She was having the eye redness from Monday."
"She's had redness in her left eye since Monday."
"You could be going for the surgery if needed."
"You may be referred for surgery depending on your progress."

RADIOGRAPHY

"I am taking your X-ray now."
"I'll take your X-ray now — it will only take a minute."
"The doctor will explain you the result later."
"The doctor will explain the results to you afterwards."

CARDIOLOGY

"You are feeling pain in the chest now?"
"Are you currently experiencing chest pain?"
"The patient was died in the ambulance."
"The patient passed away en route to hospital."

AUDIOLOGY

"You can't hearing well in the left side?"
"You're having difficulty hearing in your left ear, is that right?"
"I will make test your hearing."
"I'll carry out a hearing test to assess your range and sensitivity."

BIOCHEMISTRY

"The levels was showing abnormal."
"The results showed elevated enzyme levels."
"Maybe you are needing more test."
"You may require further testing to confirm the cause."

HAEMATOLOGY

"He didn't had the blood check last month."
"He didn't have a blood test last month."
"The bloods was taken today morning."
"The blood samples were taken this morning."

RADIOGRAPHY

"You go inside and sit for the scan."
"Please step into the scanning room and take a seat."
"The MRI it take 20 minute."
"The MRI will take approximately 20 minutes."

MICROBIOLOGY

"The bacteria was found in the urine."
"Bacteria were identified in the urine sample."
"She had taking antibiotics already."
"She had already taken a course of antibiotics."

PHYSIOTHERAPY

"You doing exercise every day?"
"Have you been doing the exercises daily?"
"It can helping your movement."
"It may help improve your range of motion over time."

TRAINER STRIP – HOW TO COACH THIS

Don't start with grammar rules. Start with clinical purpose.
Then embed grammar that matches the message.
Pair role-play with grammar recasts
Pause and edit live speech
Use flash tense drills with profession-specific cases
Make them hear the difference between Band B and Band A tense use

FINAL WORD: SPEAK & WRITE IN TIME. OR FALL BEHIND.
Clinical English isn't academic. It's accountable.

It must be:
Timed
Targeted
Trustworthy
So train your grammar like it's an IV drip.
No leaks. No confusion. Just flow.

Vault Unlocked. Book Complete. Now it's game time.
Revisit your weak spots. Repeat the drills. Redo what wasn't tactical enough.

And remember:
Band A is a decision you rehearse.
Precision is how you earn it.

MODULAR ENTRY PATHWAYS

Signposted Inside This Book for Tactical Access

Track	Entry Point
SPEAKING-ONLY	Chapter 5 → Chapter 6 → Chapter 8 → Chapter 22 → Appendix A1 / A2
WRITING-ONLY	Chapter 9 → Chapter 10 → Chapter 12 → Chapter 23 → Appendix A3 / A7
LISTENING-FIRST	Chapter 20 → Chapter 24 → Appendix A6
BAND B BOOST	Band B–version companion guide (Next Phase Launch)
TRAINER MODE	Look for Coaching Notes flagged in margins

Use these modular tracks to enter where you need help most — without losing sight of the full battlefield. Let the book meet your mission, not just follow the order.

OET INTELLIGENCE BRIEF

Structure. Scenarios. Strategy. Read Before You Test.

What You're About to Face

The OET is not just a language test. It's a clinical performance scan — designed to test whether you can operate safely, clearly, and professionally in English under pressure.

It doesn't care how well you speak English. It cares how well you use it — in a clinical moment that counts.

The Four Sub-Tests (and What's Really Being Tested)

Skill	Surface Task	Strategic Focus
Listening	Extract meaning from consultations and lectures	Filter symptoms, escalate priorities, and document details fast
Reading	Navigate short and long healthcare texts	Scan, skim, and select key clinical points with precision
Writing	Write a profession-specific letter (e.g. referral, discharge)	Prioritise what matters, exclude fluff, and deliver structured clarity
Speaking	Role-play as the professional, not the patient	Take charge, educate, reassure, redirect, and close confidently

Each skill is pressure-tested under time and context stress. There's no filler. Just function.

Who the Test is Built For

One test. 12 distinct professional paths.

Doctors (Medicine)
Nurses
Dentists
Veterinarians
Pharmacists
Radiographers
Physiotherapists
Podiatrists
Occupational Therapists
Dieticians
Speech Pathologists
Optometrists
Listening and Reading = same across professions
Speaking and Writing = tailored to your role

Delivery Modes – Choose Your Weapon

Mode	Book in Advance	Test Days	Results In	Suitability
Paper Test	24+ days	Fri & Sat	17 days	Classic format, slower feedback
Computer at Centre	7+ days	Mon–Sat	10 days	Ideal for faster results and digital comfort
OET@Home®	7+ days	Mon–Sat	6 days	Fastest option — strict tech rules apply

Note: All modes test the same skills. Only the format changes. Choose based on speed, environment, and control.

Who Accepts It?
The OET is your linguistic clinical passport. It's accepted by:
NMC, GMC (UK)
ECFMG (USA)
AHPRA (Australia)
Boards in Ireland, NZ, Canada, Singapore, and beyond
If you're heading into regulated healthcare practice, OET gets you in the room. Band A gets you hired.

Strategic Lens: OET Isn't Academic. It's Operational.
You're being assessed as a working clinician:
Can you extract what matters from chaos?
Can you structure urgency into letters?
Can you speak with authority, not apology?
Band B = competent.
Band A = trusted.

Where This Fits in Care to Talk
This brief is your structural anchor. Every strategy in this book assumes you already understand the arena. But if you needed a tactical refresher, this is it.
Use it. Annotate it. Pass it to a colleague who's treating this like another English test. (They won't make it.)

OET Test Structure & Information

OET Listening – Tactical Breakdown

What you hear isn't just audio. It's pressure. Can you filter what matters — under clinical conditions?
Duration: ~40 minutes
Format: 3 Parts | 42 Questions | Clinical Pressure Simulation

Part A – The Consultation Trap
What It Is: Two real-time consultations between a healthcare professional and a patient.
Your Task: Fill in the blanks on professional notes as you listen — live.
Why It Matters: This simulates what you'd actually do during an intake or clinical interview. No rewinding. No second chances. Either you filter fast — or you miss it.

Core Skill:
Active listening under time pressure
Clinical summarising
Extracting key symptoms, concerns, and patient phrasing

Part B – Micro-Moments in the Workplace
What It Is: Six short audio extracts (about 1 minute each) from real healthcare settings: briefings, shift handovers, or patient updates.
Your Task: One multiple-choice question per clip — no context, no fluff. Just extract and decide.
Why It Matters: You're tested on whether you can catch the tone, purpose, or next step in fast clinical interactions.

Core Skill:
Spotting nuance and intent
Distinguishing between instructions, advice, concern, or opinion

Part C – Clinical Communication at Scale
What It Is: Two longer clips — usually professional interviews, podcasts, or healthcare presentations.
Your Task: Answer six multiple-choice questions per clip, covering both detail and global meaning.
Why It Matters: This tests your ability to keep track of complex information across time, tone shifts, and idea development.

Core Skill:
Following extended discourse
Identifying purpose, position, or implications

Assessment Focus

Part	Skill Target	Marking Method
A	Note-taking from live conversation	Human marked (by trained assessors)
B + C	Meaning, inference, and decision-making	Automatically scored

You're not just being tested for "right answers." You're being assessed for:
How well you track meaning
How fast you make clinical decisions
How confidently you filter real-world audio stress

CHKZ Mindset Shift

This is not a memory test. It's a clinical clarity filter.

Hear it.
Filter it.
Write what matters.

The ones who over-listen or second-guess? Fail.
The ones who extract fast and write smart? Win.

OET Reading – Tactical Breakdown

Can you extract what matters — fast, under pressure, and without losing the plot?

Duration: 60 minutes
Format: 3 Parts | 42 Questions | 1 Chance to Think Like a Clinician

Part A – The 15-Minute Blitz

What It Is: Four short texts on a single healthcare topic — patient leaflets, information sheets, medication labels, guidelines.
Your Task: Answer 20 questions: matching, short answers, sentence completions.
Why It Matters: This is a race. You have 15 minutes to scan, skim, and select without overthinking. Designed to replicate real-world info triage.

Core Skill:

Expeditious reading
Matching facts to purpose
Reading under time-attack conditions

Part B – Workplace Snapshots

What It Is: Six brief but dense texts from clinical settings — think internal memos, protocols, emails, bulletins.
Your Task: One multiple-choice question per extract.
Why It Matters: Every text mirrors what you'd face in a shift: info that affects safety, roles, and decision-making. You need to catch the intent fast.

Core Skill:

Spotting tone, policy, or instruction
Recognising subtle detail or hierarchy
Reacting like a team player, not a slow reader

Part C – Deeper Reading, Higher Stakes

What It Is: Two longer, more complex texts drawn from research, commentaries, or professional journals.
Your Task: Eight multiple-choice questions per article.
Why It Matters: This tests your ability to read like a clinician who thinks — not just reads. You'll need to track argument flow, detect bias, and follow abstract meaning.

Core Skill:

Understanding writer's position
Recognising implied meaning or bias
Processing complex ideas under time pressure
You have 45 minutes for Parts B and C combined. Time mismanagement here = guaranteed drop in score.

Assessment Focus

Part	Skill Target	Marking Method
A	Speed scanning and precise info matching	Human marked (double-marked)
B + C	Critical reading, inference, gist	Automatically scored

You're being assessed not for memorisation, but for how well you read like a professional, not like a student.

CHKZ Mindset Shift

Reading isn't passive. It's situational awareness on paper.

You're not reading. You're processing clinical evidence in real time.
The wrong scan = the wrong call.

And in the real world? That mistake has a patient attached.

OET Writing – Tactical Breakdown

This isn't creative writing. It's clinical clarity, under time pressure, with a patient's future on the line.

Duration: 45 minutes
5 minutes: Read the case notes
40 minutes: Write the letter

Task Type: Profession-Specific Letter
Doctors write for doctors
Nurses write for nurses
Vets write for vets
No mix-and-match

Most common letter types:
- Referral
- Transfer
- Discharge
- Advice or explanation
- Complaint response (rare but possible)

Structure and Simulation
You are given:
A clinical scenario with case notes
A target reader (GP, specialist, community nurse, etc.)
A task that requires extracting, sequencing, and framing information
Then you write a formal letter — clinical, focused, and fit for function.
This isn't just about English.
It's about how you prioritise, structure, and think like a clinician in writing.

Assessment Criteria – The CHKZ Breakdown

Criterion	Tactical Definition	Scoring Insight
1. Purpose	Is the reason for the letter immediately clear — and logically expanded?	Weak candidates bury the purpose. Strong ones spotlight it in Line 1.
2. Content	Are all the right clinical details included — and are they accurate?	Band A filters out noise. Band B includes too much or misses key steps.
3. Conciseness & Clarity	Is the letter clear, sharp, and stripped of clutter?	Too much case note copying = fail. Smart summarising = Band A.
4. Genre & Style	Is the tone clinical and professional? Is the letter written for this reader?	Mismatch the tone or write casually, and you're out. This is a professional handover.
5. Organisation & Layout	Is the structure logical, readable, and prioritised?	Good paragraphing isn't decoration — it's navigation.
6. Language	Is the grammar, vocab, and punctuation accurate enough not to interfere?	Perfect English isn't required. But interference = deduction.

Scoring is double-marked by trained assessors, with reference to Band descriptors from 0–7.

CHKZ Mindset Shift

This letter isn't about you.

It's about what the next clinician needs to act fast and safely.

Every sentence must earn its place.

Every word must serve care continuation.

Edit like the reader's time is limited — because it is.

You're not just writing a letter.

You're transferring clinical responsibility — in writing, with zero margin for error.

OET Speaking – Tactical Breakdown

Real role. Real patient. Real pressure. No scripts. No second takes.

Duration: ~20 minutes
Task: 2 Profession-Specific Role-Plays

Format & Flow
Warm-Up Chat *(not assessed)*: 2–3 minutes of general, friendly talk with the interlocutor

Role-Play 1
– **3 minutes**: Read the card, prep strategy
– **5 minutes**: Conduct the role-play

Role-Play 2
– Same structure as above, different clinical context
You = the clinician
Interlocutor = the patient / carer / relative
For Veterinary Science: The interlocutor plays the animal's owner or carer
Both cards show the same background — but only you have access to your detailed task prompts.

What You're Actually Being Assessed On

The OET Speaking test has two sets of criteria:

1. Linguistic Criteria – How well do you use English?

Criterion	Band A Behaviour
Intelligibility	Pronunciation is clear, natural, and doesn't cause strain. Accent is never a barrier.
Fluency	Smooth speech with no searching pauses. You sound like a clinician in control, not a student in panic.
Appropriateness of Language	You match tone, register, and word choice to the person in front of you. No awkward jargon bombs.
Resources of Grammar & Expression	You vary your structures with flexibility and accuracy — even under pressure. Idioms and transitions show up naturally.

2. Clinical Communication Criteria – How well do you lead the conversation?
OET isn't testing bedside charm.
It's testing clinical interactional control — and you're scored across 5 domains.

Domain	What Top Candidates Do
A. Relationship Building	Greet professionally. Show warmth without losing control. Stay calm, non-judgemental, and present.
B. Eliciting the Patient's Perspective	Ask what they think. Pick up cues. Align your explanation with their actual concerns.
C. Providing Structure	Signpost clearly. Sequence logically. Guide the conversation like a clinical leader.

Domain	What Top Candidates Do
D. Gathering Information	Start open. Go closed. Clarify gently. Summarise smartly. Stay out of interrogation mode.
E. Giving Information	Check what they know. Don't talk at them — talk with them. Pause. Reframe. Confirm understanding.

Each criterion is scored from 0 to 3. You don't need to be perfect — but you must perform with consistency and professional control.

CHKZ Tactical Insight

The best candidates don't sound "fluent."
They sound professional, structured, and clinically safe — even in high-stress scenarios.

You're not being marked on accent.

You're being marked on:
Presence (tone + confidence)
Performance (task completion + clarity)
Pressure-proof delivery (no fumbles, no panic, no waffling)

CHKZ Mindset Shift
This is not "speaking practice."
It's your clinical authority test.

You're not "pretending" to be a nurse, vet, doctor.
You are one — for five minutes that count more than most of your training ever did.

Win this test by:
Staying in role
Owning the task
Keeping the patient safe and informed — in language that lands, not lectures

THE SIMULATION SUITE – PART 1

One Task. Four Skills. No Excuses.

Welcome to the Blue-Diamond Tactical Practice Zone — where we don't rehearse. We perform.

Each sub-test below includes:

1 **Full Practice Task** (modelled on OET format)
Tactical tips for Band A
Strategy drills and mindset shifts
Commentary and scoring rubrics
Trainer prompts + reflection

LISTENING – Band A Simulation
Part A: *Consultation Extract*
Audio Scenario:
A GP speaks with a 53-year-old man, Mr Salim, who has returned with worsening symptoms of fatigue and breathlessness.
Task: Fill in the doctor's consultation notes (12 gaps total).

Band A Strategy:
Listen for clinical signposts (e.g. "I've been feeling...", "It's worse when...")
Don't write full sentences — prioritise key data
Use abbreviations only if accurate (e.g. SOB = shortness of breath)
Tune in for time-based symptoms (duration, frequency)

EXAMINER TRIGGER POINT:
Clear symptom structure = Band A
Paraphrase error or omitted critical detail = Band B
Trainer Tip: Coach note-filtering under real-time replay limits. One listen only. Debrief by asking: What would a GP miss if you left this out?

Part B: *Short Workplace Extracts*
Scenario: 6 audio clips – team briefing, hospital memo, radiology update, discharge planning, pharmacy instruction, and a home visit report.
Task: 1 MCQ per clip. Choose the best answer.

Band A Strategy:
Predict what you're about to hear using the lead-in
Eliminate distractors based on function not just content
Prioritise tone and purpose (e.g. instruct, clarify, escalate)

Part C: *Presentation/Interview*
Scenario: A hospital administrator discusses infection control with a public health specialist.
Task: 6 MCQs — infer speaker opinion, purpose, emphasis.
Band A Strategy:
Listen for attitude, comparison, future plans
Avoid literal answers — go for intent and implication

Stay engaged for shifts in stance: "However...", "That said..."
Band A Marker Tip: Confident candidates infer purpose; Band B candidates stay stuck in surface detail.

READING – Band A Simulation
Part A: Expeditious Reading
Theme: "Managing Chronic Pain"
Four short texts:
Patient leaflet
Dosage chart
NHS clinical update
Over-the-counter medication table
Task: 20 questions (match, complete, short-answer)

Band A Strategy:
Scan for keywords in the question, not the text
Use headers and bullet points as scanning anchors
Don't over-read — your job is location + extraction

Part B: Workplace Extracts
Texts:
Discharge checklist
Ward infection protocol
Internal email re: documentation changes
Memo on overtime
Safety alert
Handover note
Task: 6 MCQs

Band A Strategy:
Check what's expected vs instructed
Focus on intended recipient (who is this message for?)
Look for clues in tone: "staff must vs staff are advised"

Part C: Long Articles
Title 1: "The Rise of Telehealth: Patient Risks and Gains"
Title 2: "Multidisciplinary Collaboration in Oncology Units"
Task: 8 MCQs per article (opinion, inference, tone)

Band A Strategy:
Track the writer's voice
Highlight connector words: "although," "despite," "in fact"
Don't confuse what is said with what is implied
Trainer Note: Use "quote and prove" strategy. Learner states the answer, then highlights the justification.

WRITING – Band A Simulation
Task Type: Referral Letter (Medicine)
Scenario:
You're a junior doctor at A&E. You saw Mr Brian Hunt, a 68-year-old retired builder, who presented with chest discomfort, nausea, and diaphoresis. You're writing a referral letter to the cardiology department for further evaluation.

Case Notes Include:
Social history (smoker, alcohol intake)
Vitals + ECG findings
Family history
Medication started in A&E
Follow-up needs

BAND A MODEL STRUCTURE
Paragraph 1: Clear reason for referral. Summary sentence.
Paragraph 2: Presenting complaint + acute symptoms
Paragraph 3: Past medical & social history relevant to cardiology
Paragraph 4: Action taken + suggested follow-up
Close: Clinical tone. No over-politeness. No apology or emotion.

BAND A SCORING LENS

Criterion	Band A Behaviours
Purpose	Immediately clear in opening line and justified across letter
Content	Accurate case filtering – relevant, prioritised
Conciseness	No fluff, no duplication, high signal-to-noise ratio
Style & Genre	Clinical, factual, respectful to reader role
Organisation	Paragraphed by logic, not habit
Language	Errors, if any, never impede understanding

Trainer Trick: Ask: "Would a cardiologist want to read this after a 12-hour shift?"

SPEAKING – Band A Simulation
Scenario 1: *Nurse + Post-Surgical Patient*
Patient is anxious about discharge. Role-play involves:
Explaining wound care
Clarifying medication
Addressing concern about going home alone

Band A Approach:
Open with control: "Good morning Mr Green, I understand you're being discharged today. Let's go through everything so you feel confident managing at home."

Use short, structured explanations:
→ "There are three things I want to cover   "
Check understanding:
→ "Would you like me to go over that again or is it clear so far?"

Scenario 2: *Vet + Dog Owner*
Owner brings in Bella, a 6-year-old Labrador with sudden limping. Role-play involves:
Eliciting symptoms
Explaining next steps
Managing emotional distress (child recently died; dog is all she has left)

Band A Approach:
Show empathy without derailing clinical focus

Say less, mean more:
→ "I can see how much she means to you. Let's figure out what's going on and how we can help her feel better quickly."

SPEAKING SCORING SNAPSHOT

Linguistic	Band A
Pronunciation	Clear, confident, not effortful
Fluency	Controlled speed, no filler spirals
Appropriateness	Patient-safe, no over-formality
Grammar/Vocab	Precise, flexible, clean

Clinical Communication	Band A
Relationship	Warm but focused
Eliciting	Open-ended, responsive
Structuring	Signposted, paced
Gathering	Targeted without interrogating
Giving Info	Explains, checks, adapts

Final Coaching Prompts
Listening: Can you extract under pressure — or just passively hear?
Reading: Can you process like a practitioner — or scan like a student?
Writing: Would you trust yourself with a real handover?
Speaking: Would you reassure a stranger — or just impress an examiner?

THE SIMULATION SUITE – PART 2

Second Wave. Higher Stakes. Still No Excuses.

You survived the first simulation.
Now it's time to train the edge — nuance, complexity, tone control, and critical decision points.

Each sub-test again includes:
A full advanced-level practice task
CHKZ Band A strategies
Danger zones + scoring breakdowns
Trainer prompts and psychological check-ins

LISTENING – Simulation 2
Part A: *Consultation Extract*
Audio Scenario:
A community mental health nurse speaks to a 33-year-old patient with fluctuating mood and recent non-compliance with medication.
Task: Complete the nurse's progress notes (12 gaps).
Band A Target:
Capture emotional nuance as well as clinical facts
Use terminology carefully: e.g. "low affect," "reluctant," "unreliable historian"
Don't soften serious omissions (e.g. skipped meds = risk flag)
EXAMINER TRIGGER:
Missed psychosocial risk? That's an automatic Band B.

Part B: *Short Workplace Clips*
Themes:
PPE protocol update
Staff roster change announcement
Infection rate report
Miscommunication clarification call
Family complaint call
Mobile unit relocation plan
Task: Choose the best response to 6 MCQs.
Band A Strategy:
Focus on organisational tone — not just message
Identify intent vs outcome
Watch for contrasts in verbal signals ("while this has improved… we still require…")

Part C: *Interview Clip*
Scenario:
A senior geriatrician is interviewed about challenges in dementia care and the shift toward trauma-informed approaches.
Task: 6 MCQs based on inference, tone, position.
Band A Strategy:
Tune into policy vs practice tension
Watch for complex reasoning chains ("if not X, then we risk Y")
Recognise where the speaker agrees in part but not in full

READING – Simulation 2
Part A: *Expeditious Reading*
Theme: **"Vaccination Uptake Challenges in Migrant Communities"**
Sources:
WHO bulletin
Local public health campaign flyer
SMS reminder template
News op-ed from a GP
Task: 20 matching, short-answer, completion questions
Band A Danger Zone:
Avoid bias: don't assume one text is "right"
Don't let similar phrasing distract you — scan for function, not familiarity

Part B: *Workplace Extracts*
Documents:
Staff disciplinary procedure
Electronic record access memo
Medication recall notice
Transport scheduling update
Equipment calibration report
Non-compliance email warning
Task: 6 MCQs
Band A Strategy:
Spot urgency vs advisory tone
Decode chain-of-command logic (who acts next?)
Confirm whether action is required or optional

Part C: *Long Articles*
Article 1: **"Ethical Strain and Decision Fatigue in ICU Teams"**
Article 2: "Burnout vs Moral Injury – What Healthcare Gets Wrong"
Task: 8 MCQs per article — tone, argument, perspective
Band A Target:
Track argument tension (Are they building up or breaking down?)
Decode discreet critique: Look for disagreement phrased politely
Don't confuse facts cited with the author's own belief

WRITING – Simulation 2
Task: Discharge Letter (Nursing)
Scenario:
You are the charge nurse on a stroke rehab unit. Mrs Angela Longford, a 75-year-old widow, is being discharged to her daughter's home. She has mild expressive aphasia and limited mobility. You're writing to the community nursing team.
Case notes include:
Mobility status + current supports
Aphasia management strategies
Risk of falls + home safety plan
Wound care (recent pressure ulcer)
Medication handover + community referrals

BAND A STRATEGY SNAPSHOT

Start with clear purpose: "I am writing to hand over care of Mrs Angela Longford, who is being discharged following a four-week inpatient rehabilitation stay after a left-sided stroke."

Group content by risk + action, not by how it appears in the notes

Avoid vague generalisations ("needs ongoing support" → "requires twice-daily assistance with toileting and pressure area checks")

Band A Rubric Focus:

Criterion	Reminder
Purpose	Clinical, early, expanded by end
Content	Only relevant info – no social clutter
Conciseness	No duplication, no vague phrasing
Style	Empathetic but professional
Organisation	Risk-based structure preferred
Language	Clear, legible, functional English

Trainer Tip: Ask: "Could another nurse act immediately based on this letter alone?"

SPEAKING – Simulation 2

Scenario 1: Occupational Therapist + Elderly Patient
Patient reluctant to use walking aid.

Task involves:
Eliciting resistance without confrontation
Reframing for independence, not restriction
Providing safe alternatives

Band A Control Points:
Acknowledge emotion → "You've managed on your own a long time. That matters."
Clinically lead → "My job isn't to limit you — it's to keep you moving safely."
Confirm action → "Let's try the cane today. We'll adjust as we go."

Scenario 2: Dentist + Nervous Teen
Teen needs 3 fillings and is visibly panicked. Parent is absent.

Task involves:
Calming patient
Explaining step-by-step
Managing emotional + legal boundaries of consent

Band A Moves:
Use simple metaphors: "We'll clean, patch, and polish — like fixing a cracked wall."
Invite control: "You can raise your hand at any time and I'll stop."
Avoid minimising: "I can see you're nervous. That's fair. I'll take you through everything."

Scoring Precision

Clinical Criterion	Band A Signs
Empathy	Tailored, not scripted responses
Eliciting	Fewer questions, more listening
Structure	Smooth signposting ("Let's move to…")
Info-giving	Adjusts tone, confirms understanding
Relationship	Assertive professionalism with warmth

Final Round: CHKZ Self-Coaching

What did I do that a real clinician would respect?

Did I structure for clarity or out of habit?

If I was recorded, would I be quotable — or forgettable?

THE SIMULATION SUITE – PART 3

This isn't practice anymore. This is pressure proofing.

Each of the following simulations exposes cracks — in reasoning, empathy, structure, and decision-making. Candidates aiming for Band A must now demonstrate control in complexity, not just competence in comfort.

LISTENING – Simulation 3
Part A: Consultation Extract
Audio Scenario:
A patient presents with poorly controlled type 2 diabetes, frequent urination, and recent blurred vision. The GP discusses potential complications and the patient's reluctance to take insulin.
Task: Fill in 12 gaps in the GP's notes.
Band A Focus:
Extract clinically serious details under emotional overlay
Accurately phrase patient beliefs vs clinician facts
Include timeline clues (e.g. "past 2 weeks," "worse after lunch")
Band B Risk: Paraphrasing inaccurately, skipping over sensitive resistance

Part B: Short Workplace Extracts
Themes:
Equipment ordering delays
Policy update on informed consent
Shift handover (high-risk patient flags)
Lab error correction
Verbal warning delivery
Visiting hours escalation issue
Task: 6 MCQs
Band A Strategy:
Identify subtext and hierarchy ("as per the senior consultant's instruction…")
Watch for contradictions or policy gaps
Choose answers that reflect organisational logic, not emotion

Part C: Extended Presentation
Scenario:
A health economist explains the pressures on rural emergency services and proposes remote triage hubs.
Task: 6 MCQs – intent, implications, ethical lens
Band A Strategy:
Detect the reasoning chain, not just data points
Identify when a speaker is justifying risk trade-offs
Track shifts from practical to political language

READING – Simulation 3
Part A: Expeditious Reading
Theme: "Post-operative care protocols across borders"
Sources:
International nursing journal
Hospital discharge plan
Patient-facing infographic

Training slide printout
Task: 20 rapid-response questions
Band A Target:
Extract under conflicting phrasing
Sort between instructional vs advisory tone
Recognise when data is outdated vs reaffirmed

Part B: Short Texts
Documents:
Updated CPR flowchart
Departmental email about cultural competence training
Adverse event form summary
Handwritten incident note
Meeting minutes (abbreviated)
Union bulletin about weekend coverage
Task: 6 MCQs
Band A Danger Zone:
Misreading tone of union or policy documents
Missing a subtle chain-of-responsibility shift

Part C: Long Articles
Article 1: "AI vs Human Judgement in Diagnostic Imaging"
Article 2: "Speaking Up: Why Junior Staff Still Stay Silent"
Task: 8 MCQs per article
Band A Strategy:
Spot author bias disguised as balance
Detect discomfort, not just disagreement
Track structural argument, not just opinion

WRITING – Simulation 3
Task: Transfer Letter (Physiotherapy)
Scenario:
You are a hospital-based physiotherapist writing to the outpatient rehabilitation team about Ms Karen Doyle, a 55-year-old who underwent knee replacement. She has shown strong progress but reports ongoing balance issues on stairs and is fearful of outdoor walks. No home support. Lives alone.
Case notes include:
ROM, strength, stairs progress
Current assistive devices
Home safety assessment pending
Co-existing lower back pain
History of poor rehab compliance

BAND A Priorities
Open with clinical summary + clear reason for transfer
Balance progress with residual risk
Use precise terms: "initially non-compliant; currently adherent with encouragement"
Mention psychosocial red flags without speculation
Trainer Tip: Ask the candidate: "If the outpatient team misreads this letter, what happens to the patient?"

SPEAKING – Simulation 3

Scenario 1: Pharmacist + Elderly Carer

A carer collects meds for a patient with dementia and asks about side effects she read online. You must:

Clarify calmly

De-escalate misinformation

Empathise with emotional strain of caregiving

Explain why medication changes shouldn't be made casually

Band A Strategy:

Avoid defensiveness

Redirect toward partnership: "Let's go through what she's taking and why. If we need to call the GP together, we can."

Use plain speech without sounding condescending

Scenario 2: Speech Pathologist + Parent of Autistic Child

The parent is upset that progress is "too slow" and wants to try online programmes instead. Your task:

Acknowledge frustration

Explain realistic timelines

Reframe therapy goals

Maintain clinical leadership while respecting parental concern

Band A Strategy:

Balance validation with clinical explanation

Use phrases like:

→ "We can absolutely explore other supports — but they need to align with how your child learns best."

→ "Consistency, not speed, is what builds real gains here."

Trainer + Self-Coaching Add-Ons

Decision-Point Challenge: Ask "Where did this candidate choose poorly — not speak poorly?"

Reframe Rehearsal: Take a Band B phrase and challenge them to deliver it better.

E.g., B: "You don't need to worry."

A: "It's completely valid to feel unsure — let me walk you through it clearly."

Platinum Mindset Prompt

"Am I just completing tasks — or commanding clinical trust in English?"

THE SIMULATION SUITE – PART 4

You're not being tested. You're being trusted.

This final simulation is a Band A crucible — no hand-holding, no obvious answers. Just ethical load, emotional volatility, and the need to stay sharp, structured, and safe.

LISTENING – Simulation 4
Part A: Consultation Extract
Audio Scenario:
A palliative care nurse meets with the spouse of a terminal cancer patient. The discussion includes symptom management, ethical questions around morphine use, and emotional readiness for end-of-life care.
Task: Fill in 12 gaps in the consultation summary.
Band A Strategy:
Track emotion-coded language and reframe it clinically (e.g. "He's giving up" → "expresses withdrawal and anticipatory grief")
Don't soften critical ethical content: record accurately
Respect euphemisms, but don't omit hard facts

Part B: Short Workplace Clips
Themes:
Ethical incident debrief
Delayed patient consent
Aggressive family complaint
Multi-agency meeting minutes
Budget cuts affecting service provision
Urgent recall of surgical device
Task: 6 MCQs
Band A Focus:
Decode ethical tension vs logistical instruction
Choose answers that reflect clinical safety + policy adherence
Listen for risk language: "ongoing concern," "awaiting senior review," "not documented"

Part C: Public Health Interview
Scenario:
A senior epidemiologist addresses vaccine hesitancy and how misinformation challenges trust-building in marginalised communities.
Task: 6 MCQs
Band A Insight:
Separate speaker belief from referenced views
Identify where persuasion is strategic vs scientific
Detect subtle audience-tailoring

READING – Simulation 4
Part A: Expeditious Reading
Theme: "Do Not Resuscitate (DNR) Policies in Long-Term Care"
Sources:
Facility policy doc
Medical journal letter

Patient rights info sheet

Local news editorial

Task: 20 questions — extract, match, complete

Band A Strategy:

Decode conflicting terminology

Watch for legal vs ethical framing

Match text to tone and purpose, not just phrasing

Part B: Short Texts

Documents:

Staff email on burnout leave

Risk register extract

Clinical audit snapshot

Near-miss event report

Staff feedback form excerpt

Legal disclaimer for experimental protocol

Task: 6 MCQs

Band A Tip:

Choose options that reflect accountability + awareness

Filter technical language into action logic: What happens next?

Part C: Long Articles

Article 1: "Clinician Conscience vs Organisational Policy: Who Wins?"

Article 2: "Trust Under Fire – Health Communication in the Social Media Age"

Task: 8 MCQs each

Band A Challenge:

Navigate authorial neutrality

Track ethical contradictions and concessions

Infer implications without overreaching

WRITING – Simulation 4

Task: Complaint Response Letter (Pharmacy)

Scenario:

You are a senior pharmacist responding to a written complaint from a patient's daughter. She claims that her father was given incorrect instructions for a new medication, leading to dizziness and a minor fall. Upon investigation, the error originated from unclear verbal counselling during collection.

Supporting Info Includes:

Patient record notes

Counselling checklist

Staff training logs

Fall outcome report

Medication reconciliation sheet

BAND A STRATEGY SNAPSHOT

Own the tone: professional, respectful, never defensive

Acknowledge harm without over-admitting liability

Use risk language: "We regret the impact of this incident…"

Include forward steps: "We have since revised the counselling script for this medication…"

Structure:

Acknowledgement + empathy

Summary of findings

Corrective actions taken

Contact information for escalation

Trainer Trigger: "If this landed on your desk as a hospital director — would you trust the sender's judgement?"

SPEAKING – Simulation 4

Scenario 1: Doctor + Patient Demanding Unnecessary Antibiotics

Patient is convinced they need antibiotics for a viral sore throat. The role-play requires:

Rejecting a request with care

Educating without sounding dismissive

Managing growing irritation and distrust

Band A Control Points:

"I understand why you'd ask — let's break down why they're not the right choice today."

Use analogies if helpful: "It's like using a fire extinguisher on a lightbulb. The tool doesn't match the issue."

Offer alternatives without sounding like you're compromising

Scenario 2: Physiotherapist + Underperforming Patient

A young athlete recovering from ACL surgery is frustrated by slow progress and has been skipping rehab sessions. Your job:

Address the behaviour

Motivate without sugar-coating

Rebuild the therapeutic alliance

Band A Moves:

"Frustration is normal — it means you care. But what happens next is on us both."

"The knee heals at its pace. But your progress depends on consistency — and I want that win as much as you do."

Optional Trainer Prompts

"Would a Band A clinician speak this way in front of a regulatory board?"

"Does this response build trust or just avoid conflict?"

"Is this performance persuasive, not just polite?"

Final Reflection

You're no longer preparing for a test. You're rehearsing for real leadership.

Language is no longer the barrier. Now your communication is the care.

CHKZ PHRASE BANK: BAND A vs BAND B - Speak like someone will quote you. Write like the handover matters.

This bank breaks down the difference between Band B and Band A performance — clinically, linguistically, and professionally. Use it to rehearse, upgrade, or audit any clinical exchange.

SCENARIO	FUNCTION	PROFESSION(S)	BAND B PHRASE	BAND A UPGRADE
Reassuring anxious patient	Reassurance	Nursing, Medicine	"Don't worry, it'll be okay."	"It's completely understandable to feel this way – let's go through what we can do to keep you safe and comfortable."
Explaining delay in treatment	Explanation	All	"There's a wait."	"There's a short delay while we prepare your results – I'll keep you informed every step of the way."
Refusing unnecessary antibiotics	Clinical refusal	Medicine, Pharmacy	"We can't give that to you."	"I understand why you'd ask. Based on your symptoms, antibiotics wouldn't help and could cause harm – let me explain why."
Advising post-surgical care	Instruction	Nursing, Physio	"You should rest."	"To support healing and prevent complications, I'd recommend keeping your leg elevated for the next 48 hours."
Calming a worried parent	Emotional control	Paediatrics, Allied Health	"Just calm down."	"You're clearly concerned – let me walk you through exactly what we're doing and why."
Clarifying a misunderstanding	Clarification	All	"That's not what I said."	"Let me clarify what I meant so we're completely aligned moving forward."
Closing a role-play	Ending	All	"Okay, bye."	"Is there anything else you'd like me to explain before we finish?"
Handling refusal of care	Persuasion	Nursing, Medicine	"You have to do it."	"I respect your decision. Can I share why this could be important for your recovery?"
Giving bad news	Delivery	Medicine, Oncology	"It's not good."	"I wish I had better news – the results show the condition has progressed. Let's go through what this means together."
Explaining next steps	Structuring	All	"We'll do some things next."	"**There are three key steps we'll take now**: a blood test, a scan, and a follow-up with your consultant."
Addressing medication error	Professionalism	Pharmacy, Admin	"It happened, sorry."	"We acknowledge the error and have reviewed our procedures to prevent

				recurrence. Your safety remains our top priority."
Managing aggressive tone	De-escalation	All	"You need to calm down."	"I can hear how upset you are – let's work together to get this sorted safely."
Handling cultural misunderstanding	Sensitivity	All	"That's not how we do it here."	"I understand this might differ from your expectations – let me explain how our process works and why."
Summarising care plan	Summary	All	"So, yeah, that's it."	"**To summarise**: we'll monitor your blood pressure, adjust your meds, and review in 2 days. Does that sound okay?"
Encouraging self-care	Motivation	Allied Health	"You should exercise more."	"Building activity into your routine will help with mobility and confidence – even a short daily walk makes a difference."
Informing family of discharge	Notification	Nursing, Social Work	"He's going home today."	"He's medically fit for discharge today. We've arranged follow-up care and reviewed the home setup with him."
Responding to emotional breakdown	Containment	Mental Health	"Don't cry."	"This is a lot to take in. It's okay to feel overwhelmed. I'm here with you – let's take this step by step."
Discussing end-of-life options	Ethical clarity	Palliative Care	"There's nothing we can do."	"At this point, our focus shifts to your comfort and dignity – let's talk about what matters most to you now."
Explaining test results	Communication	Radiology, GP	"The scan's fine."	"The scan shows no signs of damage, which is a positive result. Let's discuss what that means for your symptoms."
Asking about symptoms	Questioning	All	"What's wrong with you?"	"Can you tell me what symptoms you've been experiencing, and how they've changed over time?"
Dealing with non-compliance	Behavioural feedback	All	"You didn't follow instructions."	"I noticed there were some challenges with the treatment plan – can we explore what got in the way?"
Managing health beliefs	Framing	Medicine, Allied Health	"That's not true."	"I can see where that idea comes from. Let's look at what the evidence says and what we know about your condition."

Use this page:
Before role-plays or speaking prep
To rehearse phrase swaps under pressure

For trainer-led "Band Upgrade Challenges"

Reflection: Which Band B habits do I default to under stress? What's my upgrade phrase?

GLOSSARY: Terms That Matter

Cut the confusion. Own the language. Perform like a pro.

Band A
The highest scoring bracket in OET. Reserved for performance that is clear, controlled, precise, and contextually excellent. Band A is clinical leadership — not just language accuracy.

Band B
Competent and safe — but not commanding. Acceptable for many licensing boards, but not always enough for high-level placements or specialist registration.

Interlocutor
The trained OET examiner who plays the patient, carer, or client in Speaking role-plays. Not your enemy — but not your friend either. They score you silently.

Sub-Test
One of the four components of OET: Listening, Reading, Writing, and Speaking. Each one tests a different clinical communication mode under pressure.

Criterion / Criteria
The official scoring categories used by OET assessors. Each sub-test has its own. Every point you lose is traceable to one.

Clinical Control
The ability to guide a conversation or letter with confidence, appropriateness, and authority — even under pressure or when patients challenge your decisions.

Safe Language
Language that maintains clinical, legal, and emotional safety. No slang. No ambiguity. No guesswork. Examples: "I'm concerned that…" | "Let me clarify…"

Band C Trap
A common phrase or behaviour that pulls your score down. Usually vague, over-polite, off-topic, or linguistically weak under test conditions.

CHKZ
Our in-house system: Clarity, Honesty, Knowledge, Zero-Fluff. Every chapter, phrase, and strategy in this book is CHKZ-engineered for real-world and test-world mastery.

Blue-Diamond Drill
High-pressure practice activities designed to simulate OET conditions. If you sweat here, you score there.

Test Pressure
The cognitive, emotional, and time pressure candidates feel during OET. Band A performers plan for it, train with it, and speak through it.

Clinician Voice

Your test tone. It must combine clarity, care, and command. You are not a language student — you are a healthcare professional proving you belong in the system.

Upgrades

Strategic substitutions that turn weak language into scoring language. E.g., Replace "It's OK, don't worry" → with "It's understandable to feel that way — let's go through the next step together."

Vault

Companion digital resources provided via QR code or download link. Includes printable templates, extended drills, self-scoring tools, and bonus materials by profession.

Simulation Suite

A section in this book that includes one full example task per sub-test (L/R/W/S) — with model answers, commentary, and scoring strategy.

Profession-Specific

Tasks and scenarios designed for your exact field — e.g., dentistry, dietetics, veterinary science — not generic ESL tests.

Trainer Strip

Coaching margin notes embedded in chapters. Designed to support peer feedback, tutor guidance, and self-improvement.

Real-World Transfer

The way OET skills improve your actual clinical communication. If your test language wouldn't work in a real consultation, it doesn't belong in your OET either.

Strategic Reframe

A mental or linguistic shift that puts you back in control. Used in both Speaking and Writing to handle pressure moments.

AUTHOR'S NOTE

Thank you.

From one professional to another, thank you for choosing to engage with this book — not as a passive resource, but as a performance manual for reclaiming clarity, credibility, and control in clinical communication.

This guide was never designed to be a soft landing. It was built to sharpen your thinking, pressure-test your habits, and elevate your approach to the OET — and beyond. If at any point this book caused you to pause, shift your strategy, or upgrade your mindset, then it's done its job.

Because this isn't just a test. It's a threshold.

A threshold between:
– Band B and Band A.
– Confusion and confidence.
– Speaking to get through... and speaking to lead.

Your decision to train at this level speaks to the kind of clinician you already are — or are becoming. One who understands that communication isn't decoration — it's clinical safety, trust, and power in action.

If this guide has helped you refine your performance, reframe your standards, or remind yourself why your voice matters, then I invite you to do one thing:

Keep going.
Sharpen others.
Raise the bar — not just for the test, but for the system you'll be working in.

To continue the journey, explore companion resources, or join our next-level training, visit www.chkz.uk.

With strategic respect and professional solidarity,

Carl Halford
Author, Educator, Clinician Ally

ABOUT THE AUTHOR

Carl Halford is an educator, entrepreneur, and leader who has spent his career challenging the norm, disrupting the status quo, and demanding better. With experience spanning multiple countries, industries, and roles, he has worked as a healthcare worker, psychiatric nursing assistant, mortuary technician and manager, a teacher, headmaster, business owner, coach, and mentor—dedicating his life to empowering people to think critically, lead boldly, and break free from outdated systems.

His professional journey has taken him across the UK, Russia, Germany, China, Vietnam, Iraq, Algeria, and Georgia—where he has led teams, built businesses, and, yes, failed spectacularly in some, only to rise stronger each time. Through these experiences—both the wins and the wipeouts—he has developed a deep understanding of education, leadership, entrepreneurialism, decision-making, and resilience.

Carl believes that real education isn't about memorisation—it's about mastery, adaptability, and independent thought. *His work, his writing, and his teaching all centre around one mission*: to help people unlearn the nonsense they've been conditioned to accept and reclaim their ability to think for themselves.

When he's not writing, teaching, or leading, you'll find Carl deep in business. He believes that the right education—not just the formal, institutional kind, but the kind that builds resilience, competence, and real-world intelligence—is the key to unlocking human potential.

For insights, resources, and unapologetically blunt truths about education, leadership, and life, visit www.chkz.uk.

YOUR JOURNEY (OUR JOURNEY) DOESN'T HAVE TO END HERE

Thank you for reading *Care to Talk*. If the stories, perspectives, insights, and pearls of wisdom in this book have resonated with you, then I am delighted. But this is just the beginning—your journey of growth, leading, learning, and challenging continues.

As a professional teacher, life coach, psychotherapist, international school principal, public speaker, and most importantly, a fellow human being navigating life's ups and downs in and around education, I am deeply committed to helping others unlock their potential and find meaning in their own experiences. Whether you're seeking personal growth, professional development, or simply a fresh perspective,

I'm here to support you.

Here's How We Can Stay Connected:

1. Explore My Services
If you're ready to take the next step in your personal or professional journey, I offer one-on-one coaching and psychotherapy sessions tailored to your unique needs. Together, we can work on turning your challenges into opportunities and your failures into wisdom. Visit www.chkz.uk to learn more.

2. Join My Community
Stay updated on my latest projects, workshops, and insights by following me on [social media platform(s)] or subscribing to my newsletter. Let's continue this conversation and grow together.

3. Share Your Thoughts
Your feedback means the world to me. If this book impacted you in any way, I'd love to hear about it. Please consider leaving a review on [Amazon/Goodreads/other platforms]. Your words not only inspire me but also help others discover this book.

4. Bring Care to Talk to Your Network
If you know someone who could benefit from the words in this book—whether it's a friend, family member, or colleague—I encourage you to share it with them. Sometimes, the right book at the right time can make all the difference.

5. Invite Me to Speak or Collaborate
As a public speaker, international school principal, life coach, and psychotherapist, I am available for speaking engagements, workshops, and collaborations. Whether you're hosting an event, organising a conference, or looking for a guest speaker to inspire your team or community, I'd be privileged to bring the message of *Care to Talk* to your audience.

Feel free to reach out via carl@chkz.uk or www.chkz.uk

Other Books by The Author

Fail Smart – A bold manifesto on the power of failure as a catalyst for growth. This book challenges conventional thinking, showing how setbacks can be leveraged for learning, resilience, and ultimate success. https://amzn.eu/d/2kxiJKj

Grumpy, And Proud – A candid, humorous, and unapologetic reflection on embracing one's inner curmudgeon. This book celebrates the wisdom of experience, the freedom of speaking one's mind, and the value of standing firm in a world obsessed with people-pleasing. https://amzn.eu/d/2BrgZJM

Dumb by Design – A cutting critique of the modern education system, exposing how it suppresses ambition, critical thinking, and real-world preparedness. This book calls for a radical transformation in teaching, learning, and leadership. https://amzn.eu/d/d2xPTMK

Schools Aren't Startups – A reality check for education reformers who attempt to run schools like tech startups. This book explores why quick-fix, business-driven models fail in education and what truly works in building sustainable, effective learning environments. https://amzn.eu/d/iF4Ofl2

Oliver's Story – A compelling historical romance that takes readers on a journey of love, growth, and self-discovery. Through Oliver's struggles and triumphs, this novel explores resilience, destiny, and the pursuit of meaning. https://amzn.eu/d/iLasIO4

Fake It, Take It, and Make It - A darkly motivational blueprint for outsmarting limits, owning your ambition, and turning audacity into advantage. This book is your unapologetic guide to playing bold, rising fast, and making it count. https://a.co/d/1RtSHxv

While You Slept, They Took Over - a brutal wake-up call for teachers and school leaders trapped in performative busyness and professional autopilot. With wit, wisdom, and a 0430 battle plan, this book arms you to reclaim 546 hours a year and lead with unapologetic clarity, edge, and purpose. https://a.co/d/58OZF0a

Youth Is Wasted On The Youth - a no-holds-barred manifesto that drags the truth into the light, slaps the delusion out of your screen-soaked mind, and rebuilds your worldview brick by brutal brick. It's the unapologetic blueprint for young people, parents, teachers, and coaches who are done playing nice and ready to raise lions, not lambs. https://amzn.eu/d/5B5Odxk

Grit to Glory - it's a mirror, a weapon, and a wake-up call. With 61 punch-packed chapters, it arms you with brutal truths, unshakable principles, and blueprint-style strategies to master your mindset, discipline your habits, and lead the life you were born for — no fluff, no apologies, just forward. https://a.co/d/1QShkOO

Outstanding by Design - the ultimate reboot for Cambridge teachers—equipping educators with mindset, mastery, and mission to transform lessons, inspire learners, and lead with legacy. This is your full-throttle upgrade to Cambridge excellence, classroom impact, and unapologetic educational leadership. https://amzn.eu/d/buhHIob

First Words, First Care (CEFR A1–A2) – Level 1: A complete beginner-level Medical English book designed for frontline staff, interns, and support workers in hospitals and clinics. Covers greetings, forms, basic questions, and polite workplace communication—perfect for first steps into healthcare English. https://amzn.eu/d/0cvXwf9

Comfort Through Conversation (CEFR B1) – Level 2: This intermediate-level book helps medical staff build confidence in handling patient interactions, complaints, and instructions. Ideal for nurses, carers, and reception staff who need to speak clearly, calmly, and competently in daily situations. https://amzn.eu/d/gd7HcQF

Explain to Empower (CEFR B2) – Level 3: A professional-level resource for teaching medical explanations, procedures, and patient education with clarity and accuracy. Perfect for clinicians and trainers preparing learners for real-world conversations and confident communication. https://amzn.eu/d/8hNEkRg

The Language of Leadership in Medicine (CEFR C1) – Level 4: An advanced-level book for senior nurses, trainers, and healthcare professionals navigating high-stakes clinical communication. Covers leadership, ethics, intercultural dialogue, and crisis language for those ready to lead with words that matter. https://amzn.eu/d/2j61vx7

Character Over Curriculum: the bold, brutally honest PSHE blueprint for schools and youth leaders who dare to teach identity, ambition, and integrity louder than grades or filters. With 36 catalytic chapters, it's a full curriculum reboot that rebuilds character from the inside out — for the ones who refuse to shrink to fit. https://amzn.eu/d/iod1nU8

1SiB: One School in a Book is the definitive step-by-step manual for founding a purpose-driven, Cambridge-aligned school from the ground up. From land selection to inspection readiness, it equips educational entrepreneurs with every tool, policy, and framework needed to build a school that lasts. https://amzn.eu/d/1xOGUb0

Speak to Move is a powerful 4-level English series designed for global logistics professionals. From beginner to leader, it equips learners with the language to operate, instruct, and lead with confidence across borders. https://a.co/d/7Ap1X8O

Detention Level Jokes: A darkly hilarious survival guide for educators — loaded with skits, fake CPD, and jokes they'll never put in the staff bulletin. Read it when the Wi-Fi goes down and your soul gives up. https://a.co/d/dgWQUjo

Love, Lust, Lies: A soul-stripping, raw manifesto for those done performing for love, acceptance, or peace. Love. Lust. Lies. dismantles the masks we wear and helps readers reclaim the truth they were never allowed to speak. https://a.co/d/3xrLFOD

Eye on the Patient: A Veterinary Introduction to Ophthalmology: A practical, motivational introduction to veterinary ophthalmology for students, new vets, and general practitioners. Eye on the Patient is Book One of the Veterinary Ophthalmology Trilogy—designed to inspire clinical confidence and elevate everyday eye care. https://a.co/d/9fzdQb9

The Veterinary Ophthalmology Blueprint: A Clinical and Surgical Handbook for Practitioners (Book Two): A definitive guide for veterinary clinicians navigating the complexity of eye care in practice. From diagnostics to surgery, this book delivers structure, clarity, and confidence at every clinical turn. https://a.co/d/8dCTxRr

The Surgical Eye is your clinical and procedural blueprint for mastering ophthalmic surgery. From mindset to mastery, it equips vets, trainers, and teams with the skills, SOPs, and theatre tools that matter most. https://a.co/d/3IEPOx6

Echoes From The Edge: A funeral for mediocrity. Echoes from the Edge is your final warning shot from the future—you either rise now or rot forever. https://a.co/d/5eBagPZ

The Silence Between the Sentences is not a book of poems—it's a resurrection disguised as a collection. Where ambition burns out, grief carves deep, and grace fights back, this book cuts, confronts, and rebuilds. https://a.co/d/dJkzzXh

Born to Command: A brutally honest teen leadership playbook that combines street-sharp psychology with school-aligned principles. Born to Command helps teens turn silence into strength and uncertainty into unshakable influence. https://a.co/d/ay92yuM

Teacher Fuel – CPD 101 Blueprint: The ready-to-use CPD blueprint for schools that want to build powerful teachers and powerful culture. 56 career and CPD conversations to transform the staffroom — and the learning. https://amzn.eu/d/1P2U5JB

Blue Diamond Empire Thinking: A global blueprint for building leadership-first schools, networks, and education movements that outlast trends and shape markets. Blue Diamond Empire Thinking is the definitive model for leaders ready to build and scale What Comes Next. https://a.co/d/0ORso9m

Energy English – Oil, Gas & Energy – (L1-4 CEFR A1-C1): Complete Edition (Levels 1-4) is the all-in-one training system for English across the global energy industry. With just under 1600 pages and full model answers, it transforms English from classroom theory into jobsite reality. https://amzn.eu/d/fG3dPpZ

Energy English – First Words, First Care: Level One (A1–A2) is the foundation course (Book 1) for safety-focused, real-world English in the energy sector. With 24 CEFR-aligned lessons and full model answers, it builds immediate confidence for new learners in high-risk workplaces. https://amzn.eu/d/9CZThhU

Energy English – Comfort Through Conversation (B1) is Book 2 in the Energy English series — designed to help intermediate learners lead toolbox talks, follow safety checklists, and speak clearly in daily site situations. Includes 24 CEFR B1 lessons with full model answers and industry-ready communication tools. https://amzn.eu/d/fyvz2MD

Energy English – Explain to Empower (B2) is Book 3 in the Energy English series, designed for professionals who need to explain faults, lead handovers, and deliver updates with confidence. Featuring 24 CEFR B2 lessons and full model answers, it trains the language of control, trust, and technical fluency.   https://amzn.eu/d/g04h9yi

Energy English – The Language of Leadership in Energy (C1) is Book 4 of the Energy English series — built for supervisors, auditors, and site leaders managing teams, meetings, and crises in English. With 24 CEFR C1 lessons and full model answers, this is English for command, clarity, and control. https://amzn.eu/d/b2qpQ8h

Storm Season: A brutally honest, life-saving survival manual for teens. Storm Season helps young people navigate mental storms, emotional traps, family tension, and social chaos with the tools no one else gave them. https://amzn.eu/d/d05v78m

The Deal Changed. I Didn't: This is the book for anyone who stayed loyal to an agreement that someone else silently rewrote. Whether you were ghosted, gaslit, discarded, or demoted in someone's priorities, this book is not about moving on — it's about seeing clearly.

Notes:

#CraftedToConvert
#WordsThatWork
#CopyWithImpact
#StoryToSuccess
#PenToProfit

https://paypal.me/CarlHalford

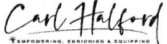

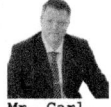

Mr. Carl
Principal & Executive CEO

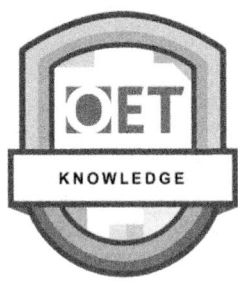

Preparation Provider: OET Knowledge

Issued by OET

The Knowledge badge covers three modules that are delivered through the Occupational English Test (OET) Preparation Provider Programme: Induction, OET Overview, and OET Knowledge. The advantage of OET (i.e. embedded in the healthcare context) and the need to improve test taking and language skills are described. The final module covers the format and skills in each sub-test and tips to help students.

Learn more

Blank Page

Blank Page

FINAL PAGE – CHKZ BACK-PAGE MANIFESTO

You weren't born to pass a test.

You were born to lead.

And the way you speak is the way you're remembered.

This book was your training.

Now go speak like you belong there.

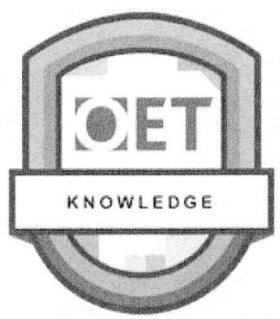

Printed in Dunstable, United Kingdom